COMMON FACIAL DERMATOSES

COMMON FACIAL DERMATOSES

RONALD MARKS

MB, BS (Hons), BSc (Hons), MRCP, DTM & H

Senior Lecturer in Dermatology,
Department of Medicine,
The Welsh National School of Medicine,
Cardiff

BRISTOL
JOHN WRIGHT & SONS LTD.
1976

ISBN 0 7236 0379 0

Printed in Great Britain by John Wright & Sons Ltd., at the Stonebridge Press, Bristol

CONTENTS

FOREWORD

'One Bardolph, if your Majesty know the man, his face is all bubuckles, and whelks, and knobs, and flames o' fire.'

Henry V, iii. vi.

The facial skin participates in many of the generalized eruptions but because of its anatomical and physiological properties it is peculiarly susceptible to changes which are unique. Being exposed to the elements as well as to the commercial enterprise of cosmetic forces it is at risk in other ways. Because the facial appearance is of such great psychosocial importance its diseases and its vagaries are inextricably tangled in both lay and medical minds with a mystique and folklore difficult to discredit.

Dr Ronald Marks has made special studies of several specific facial eruptions and is especially well placed to compile an authoritative text on this aspect of regional dermatology. Where icons are ready for destroying he is the one to topple them, where new facts have emerged Dr Marks presents them in a thoroughly concise manner.

This is indeed a sensible book and will be of equal value to General Practitioners and Specialists.

S. C. GOLD

INTRODUCTION

In the period 1965–8 I was enthralled by rosacea. In this period of study and research it became increasingly obvious to me that amidst our almost complete lack of understanding of many common skin conditions, dermatologists pontificated most and knew least about many common rashes affecting the face. Because of the lack of investigative work in either the experimental or the clinical sense the same untruths and half-truths were passed on from book to book until they became mystically enshrined by the frequency of their repetition. It seemed to me that a book devoted to common diseases of facial skin would at least serve the purpose of focusing attention on this important aspect of dermatology and our profound ignorance in this area. I felt that if I could maintain a 'critical eye', I might be able to produce something that would stimulate those who were tempted to turn the pages of a book dealing with the face. I don't know whether I've succeeded in this aim. I hope that I have and also that I have delineated the way that the face is special for dermatologists. If at times I have included subjects that are less than common I plead infatuation with things facial and would point out that 'common' is a comparative term!

It should be stated that some subjects have been dealt with in much more detail than others. Rosacea and acne have been dealt with in some detail because of my continued interest in these disorders. I trust that I have not been too skimpy with the other topics considered.

I hope that the book will be of interest not only to all practising dermatologists but to others as well, such as cosmeticians, to whom facial skin is important.

Cardiff, April 1976   R. MARKS

ACKNOWLEDGEMENTS

I wish to record my sincere gratitude and indebtedness to Dr C. B. Bentley-Phillips, without whose assistance in all the nasty details of manuscript preparation this book would never have been finished. His help and forbearance have been magnificent. I am grateful to my colleagues for encouragement and continuing to show me patients with facial rashes.

I am also grateful to the departments of Medical Illustration at the Institute of Dermatology, London, and the Welsh National School of Medicine for all the kindness and help they have given.

Lastly, I would like to express my extreme gratitude to Mrs Christine Higgins and Mrs Joy Hayes for their sterling work on an unmanageable manuscript.

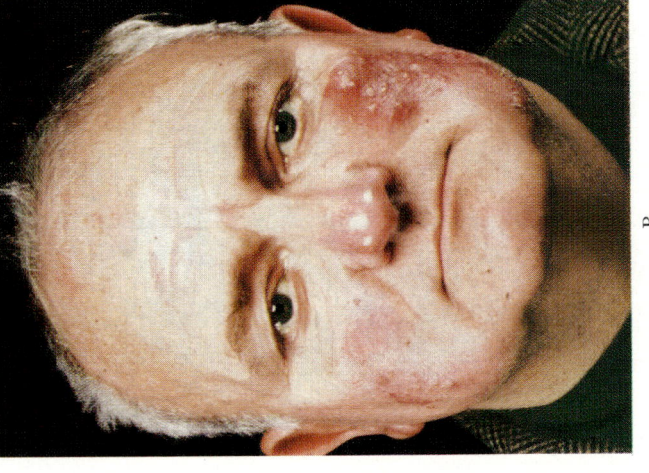

A

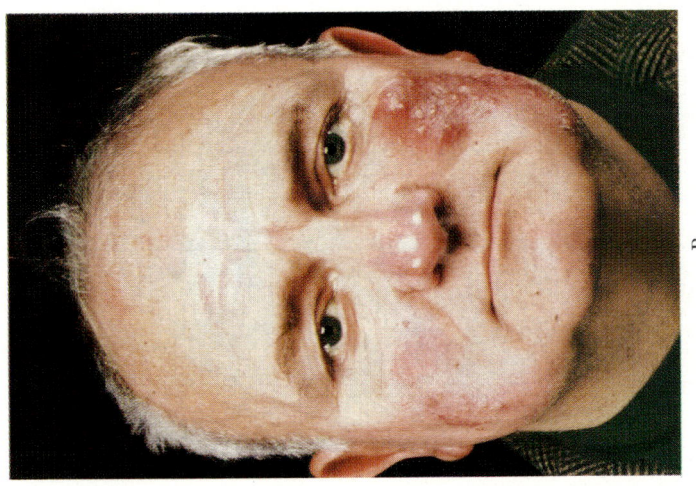

B

Plate 1.—A, Typical rosacea. B, Rosacea showing marked predilection for one side.

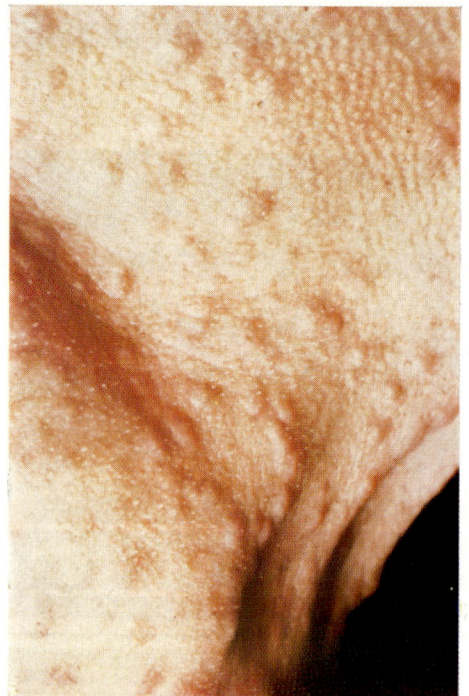

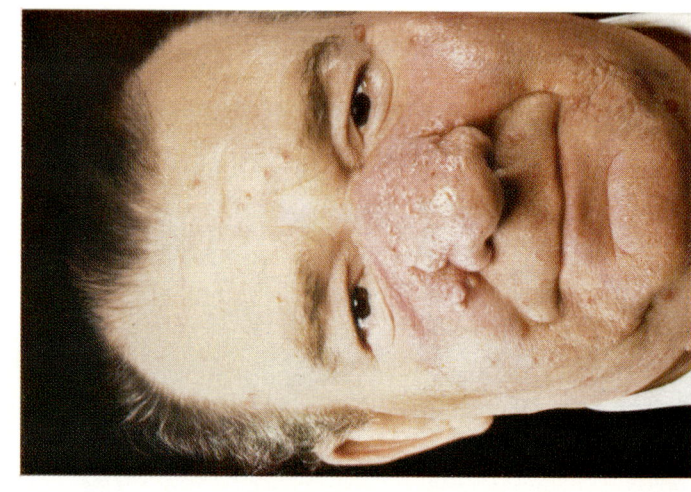

A

B

Plate 2.—A, Typical dome-shaped rosacea papules. B, Advanced rhinophyma.

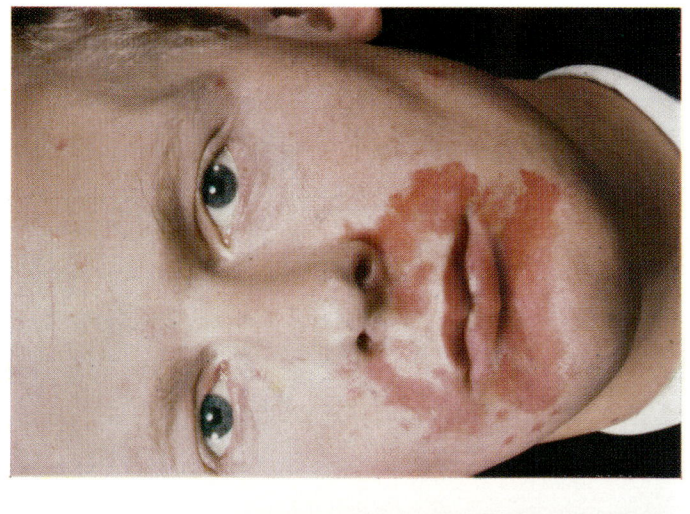

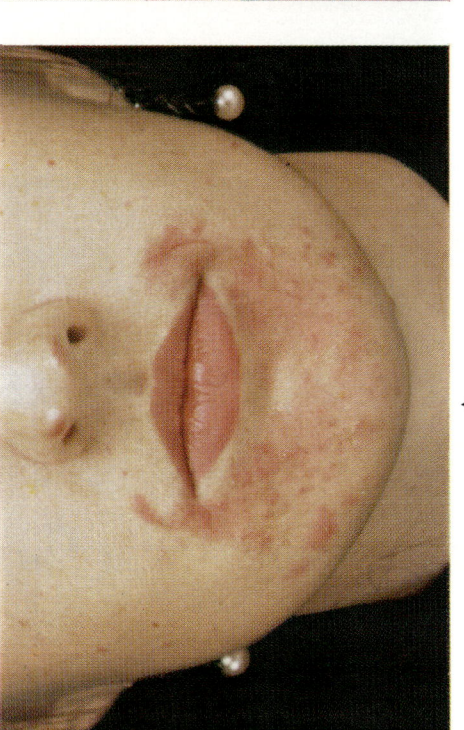

A

B

Plate 3.—A, Typical perioral dermatitis. B, Severe perioral dermatitis in a man.

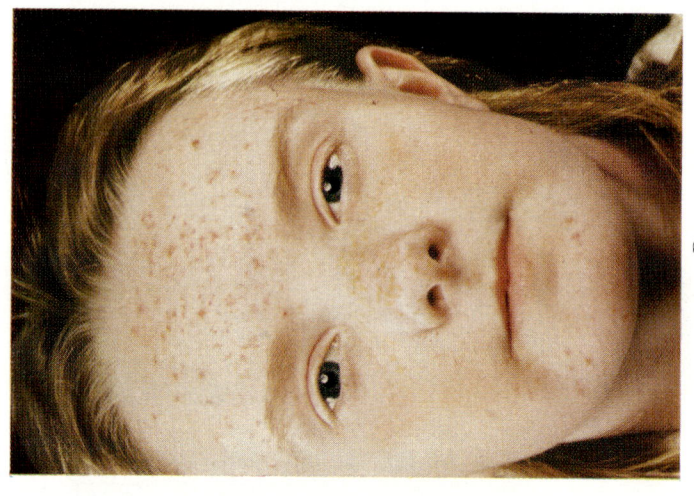

A

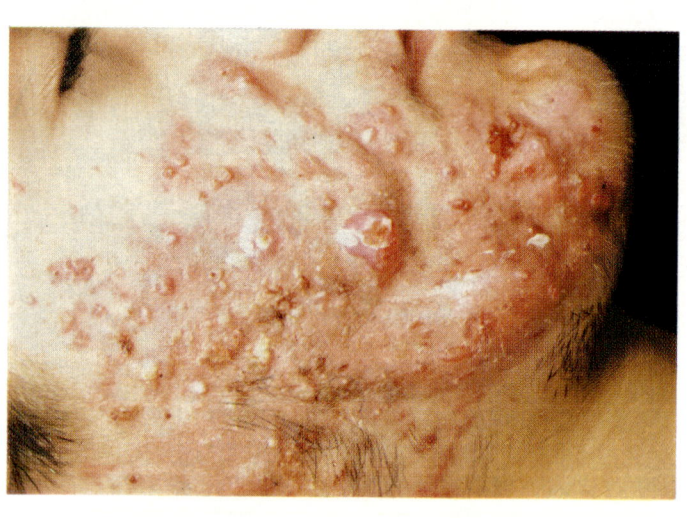

B

Plate 4.—A, Severe cystic acne. B, Mild superficial acne with blackheads, pustules and small papules.

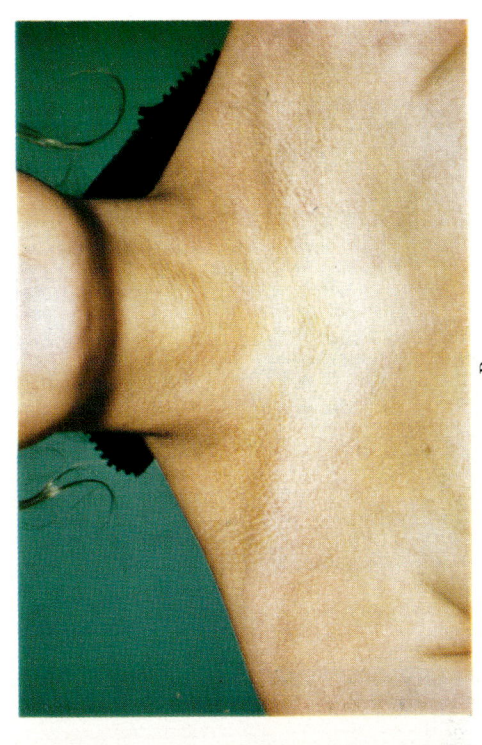

B

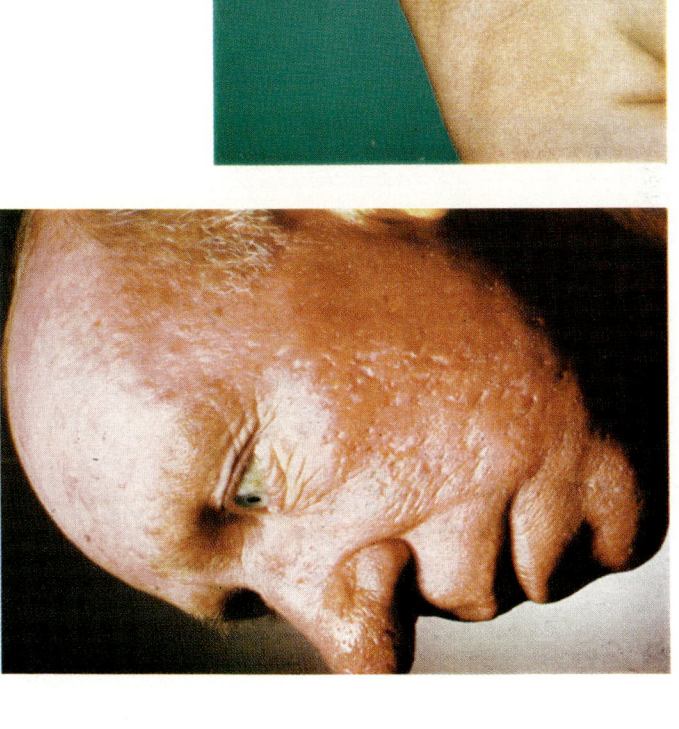

A

Plate 5.—A, 'Red acne': acne with a background of erythema—not true rosacea. B, Long-standing atopic dermatitis with pigmentary changes around the neck.

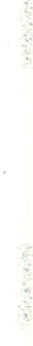

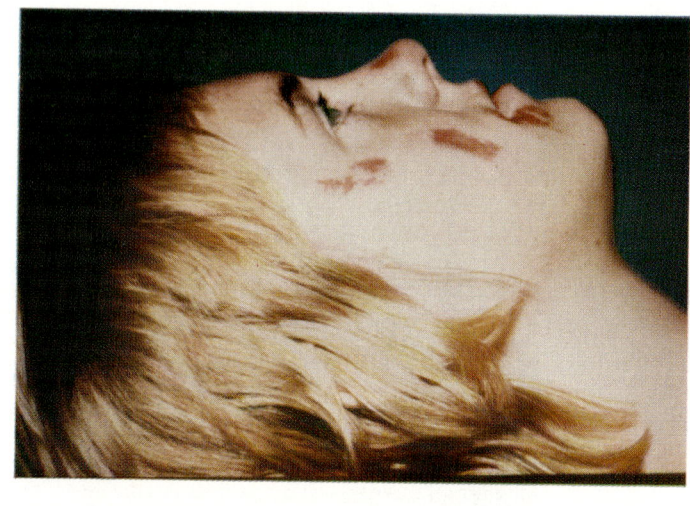

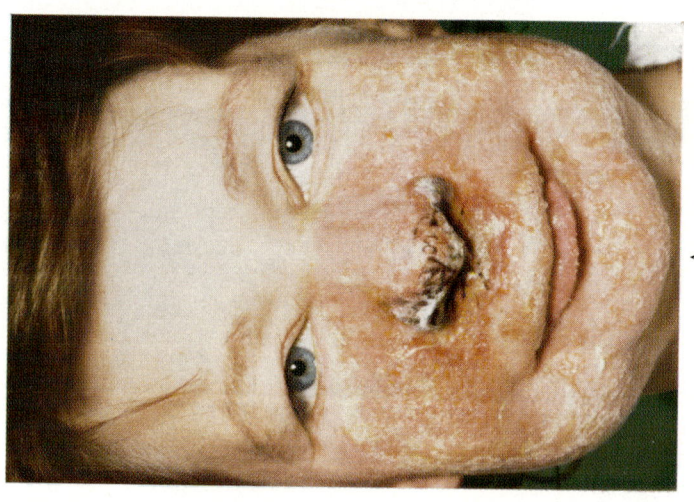

Plate 6.—A, Severe acute dermatitis of the face caused by contact hypersensitivity to chloramphenicol. B, Dermatitis artefacta.

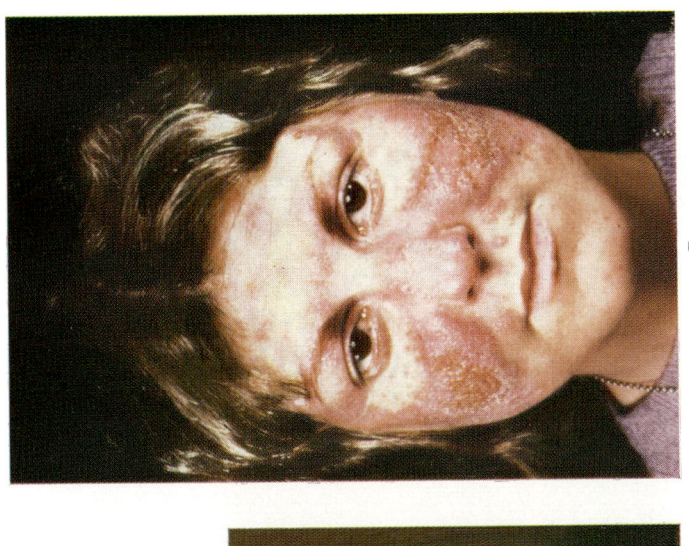

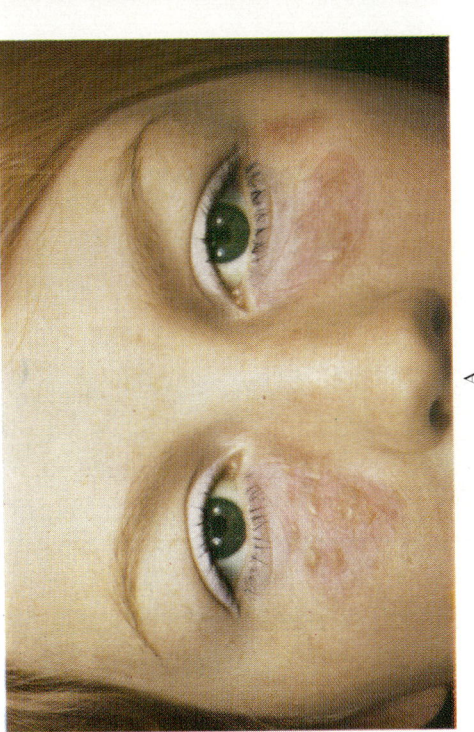

B

A

Plate 7.—A, Lesion of discoid lupus erythematosus. B, Acute systemic lupus erythematosus.

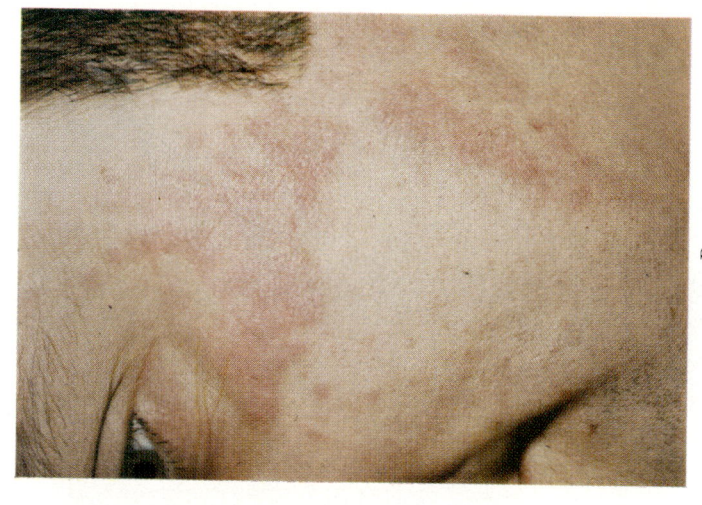

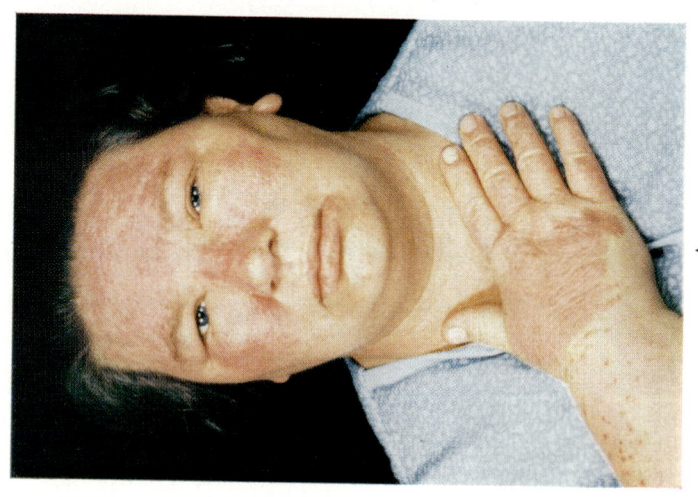

A

B

Plate 8.—A, Photodermatitis from sulphonamides. B, Jessner's lymphocytic infiltration.

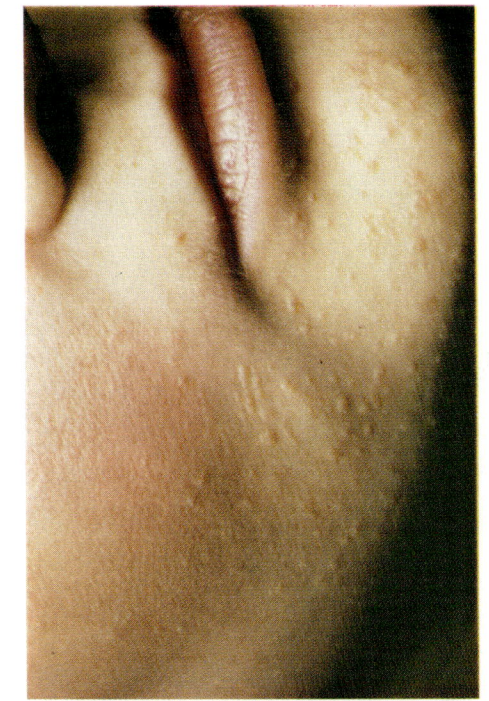

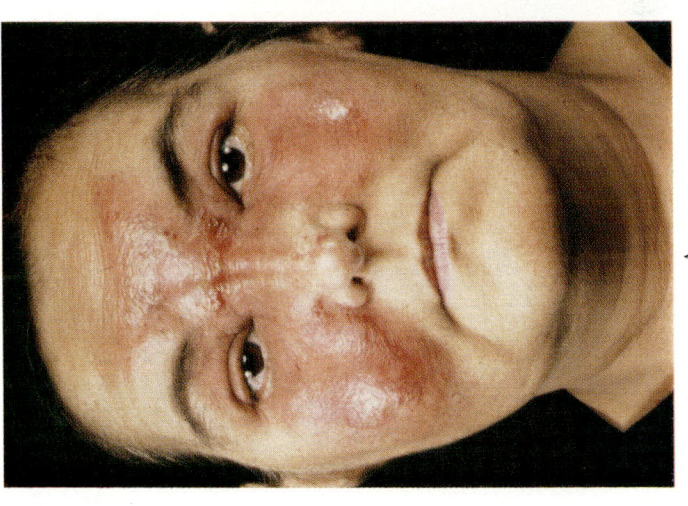

Plate 9.—A, Erysipelas of the face. B, Prolific plane warts of the face.

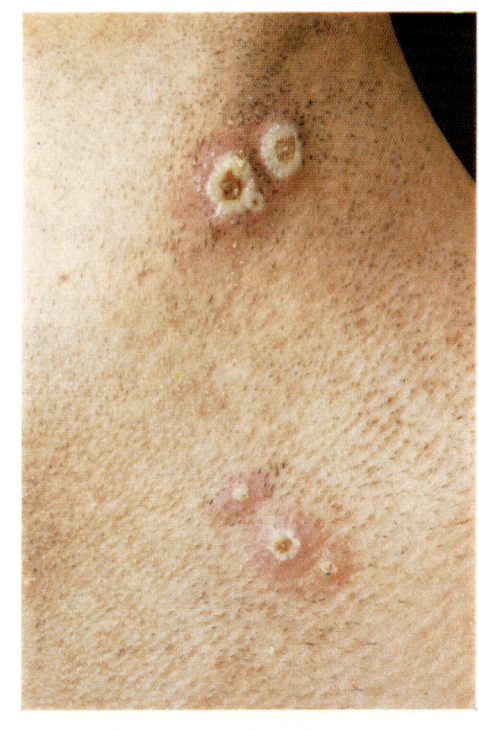

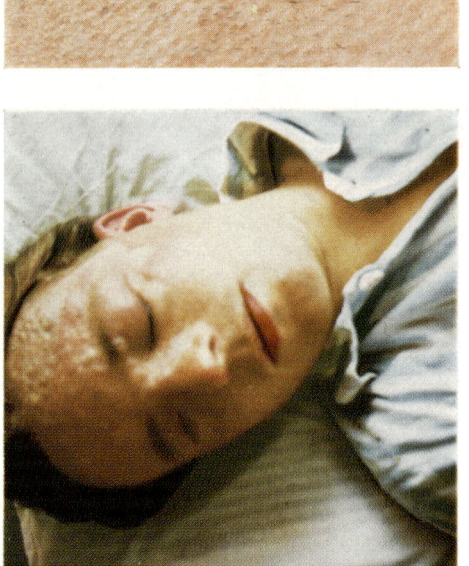

B

A

Plate 10.—A, Herpes zoster affecting ophthalmic branch of fifth cranial nerve. B, Accidental vaccinia of the neck and jaw line.

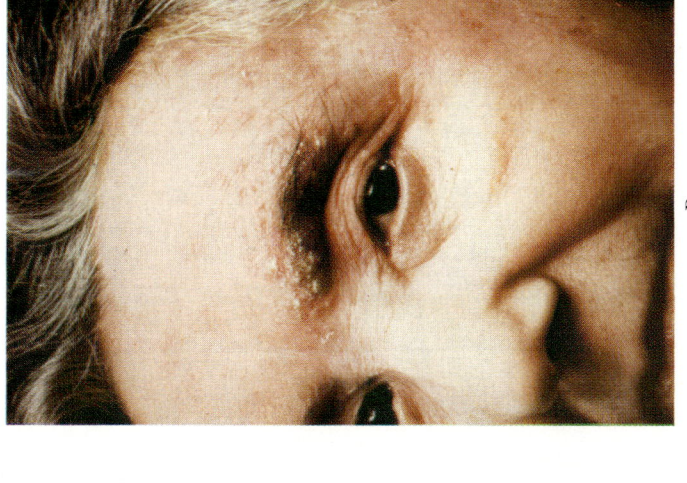

B

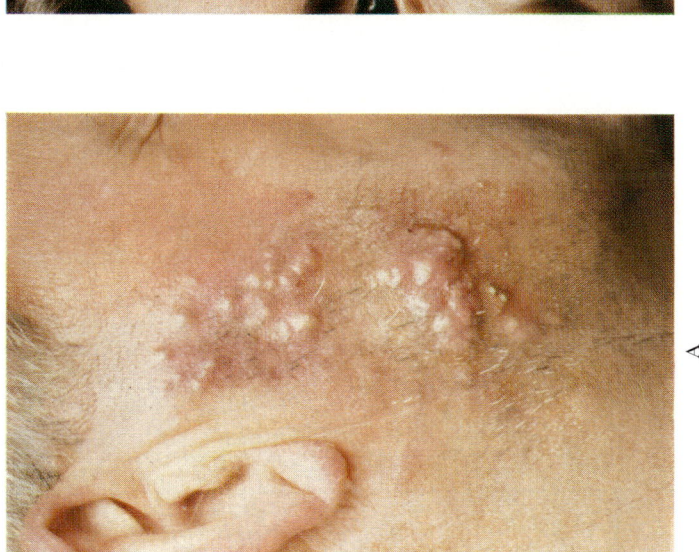

A

Plate 11.—A, Tinea barbae—this patient had been treated with topical corticosteroids. B, Steroid modified ringworm of the face—Tinea incognito.

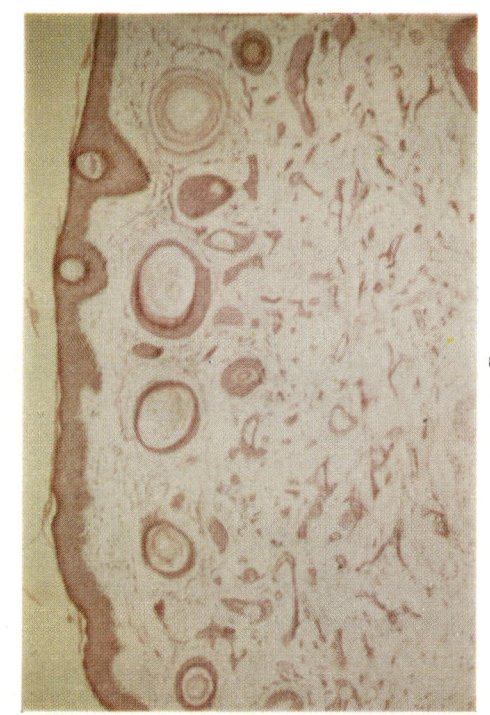

B

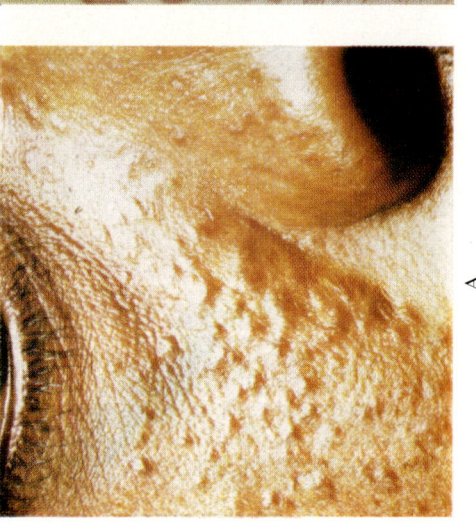

A

Plate 12.—A, Syringomata affecting the face. B, Histopathology of syringoma.

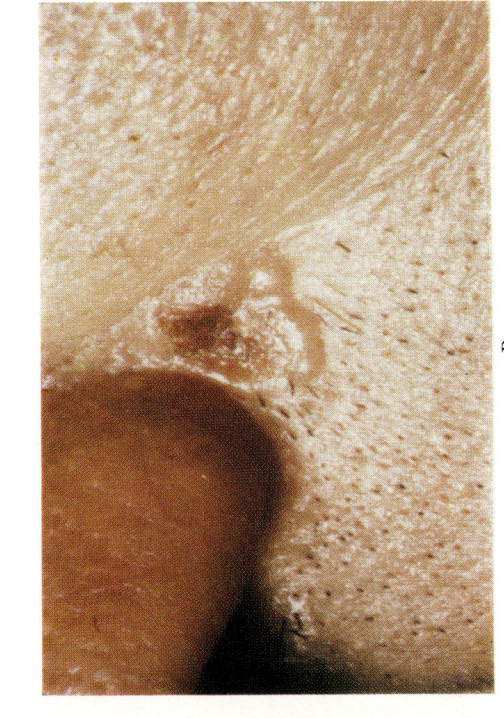

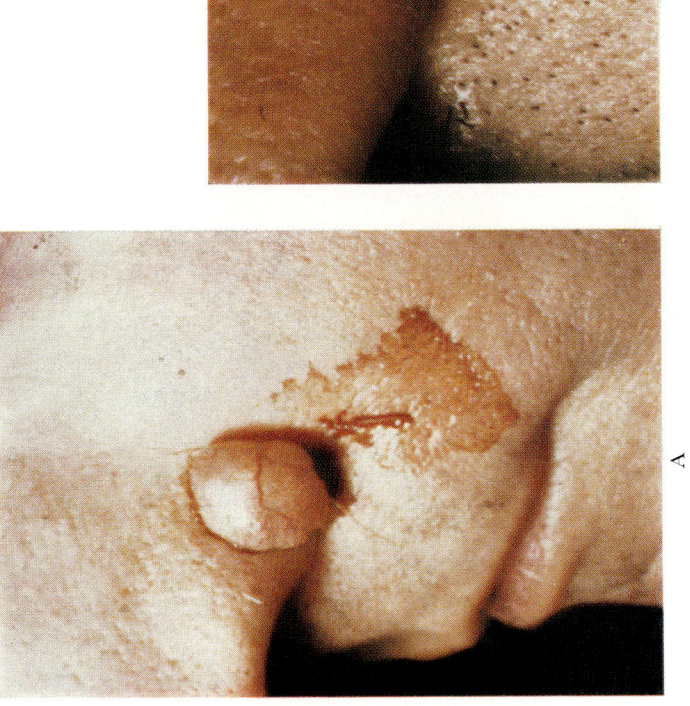

A

B

Plate 13.—A, Typical nodulocystic type of basal cell epithelioma. B, Ulcerated basal cell epithelioma.

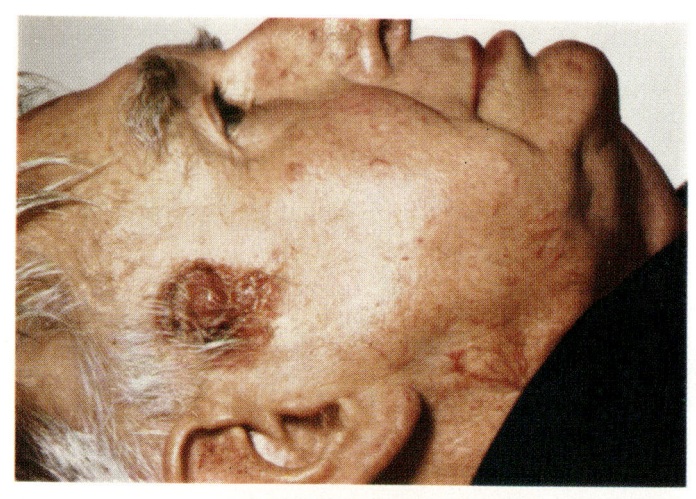

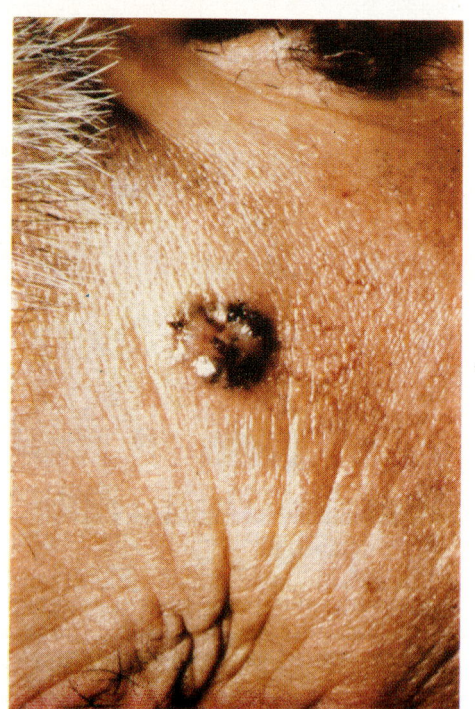

A

B

Plate 14.—A, Pigmented basal cell epithelioma. B, Squamous cell carcinoma.

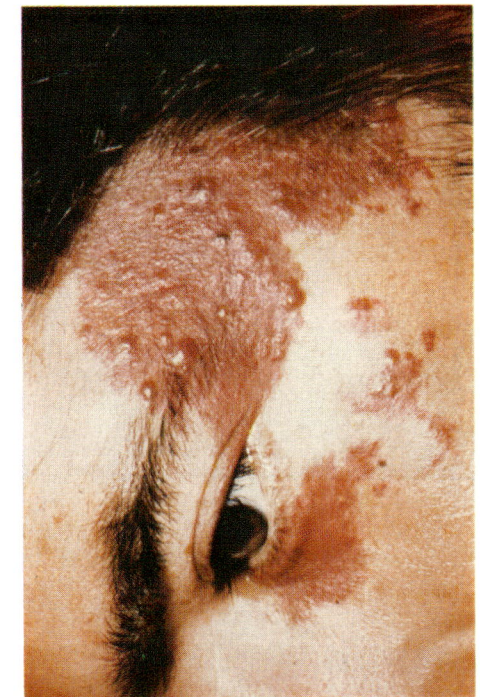

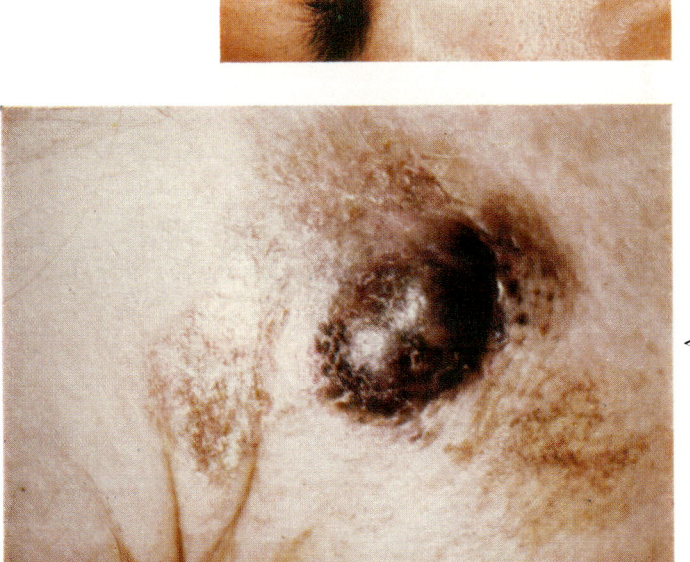

B

A

Plate 15.—A, Malignant melanoma of face. B, Extensive port wine stain.

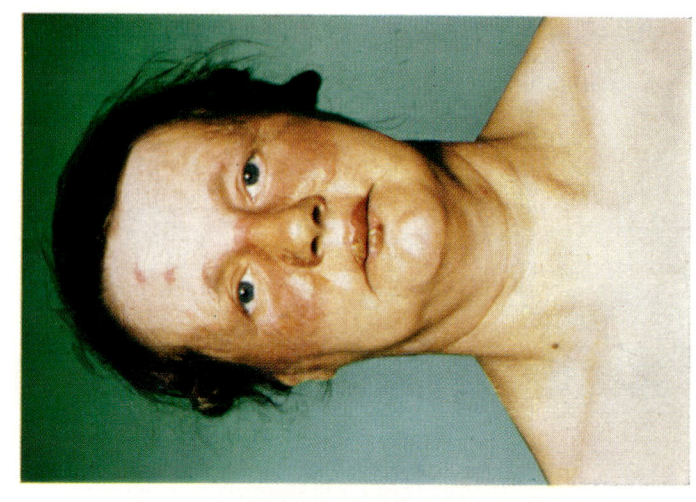

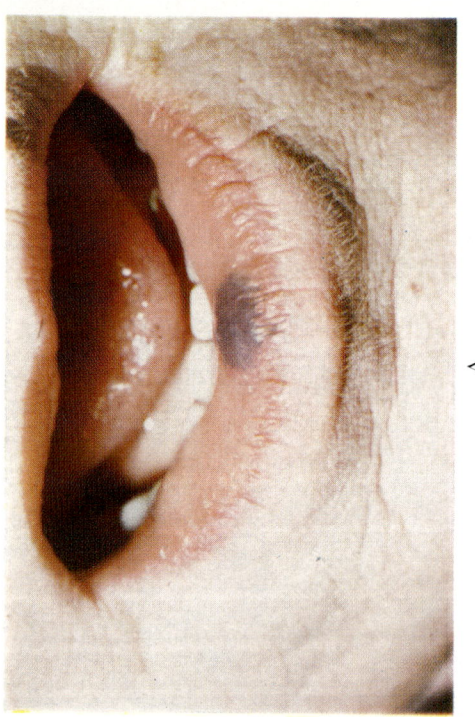

A

B

Plate 16.—A, Venous lake on lips. B, Acute febrile neutrophilic dermatosis (Sweet's disease).

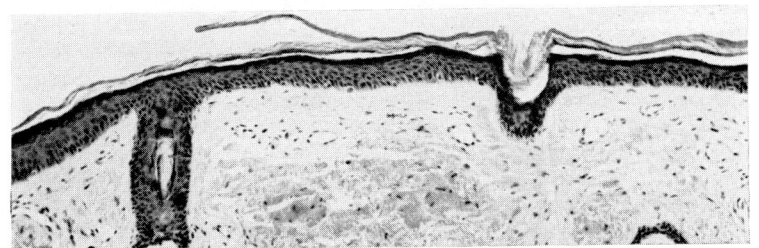

Fig. 1.—Histological section of biopsy from cheek of man of 35 showing a markedly flattened dermo-epidermal junction. There is also marked solar elastosis in the dermis. (HE; ×22.)

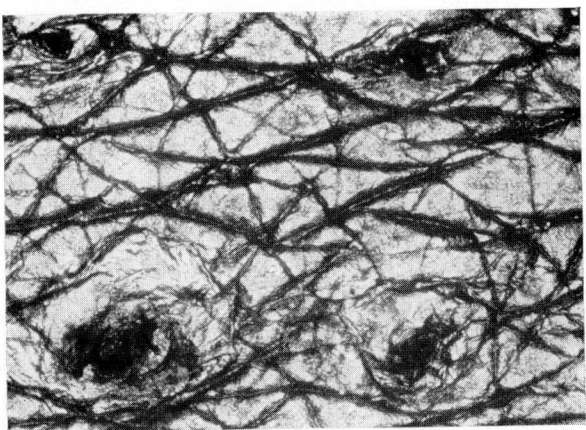

Fig. 2.—Skin surface biopsy from beard area of young man showing prominent hair follicle openings and skin markings. (Unstained; ×7·5.)

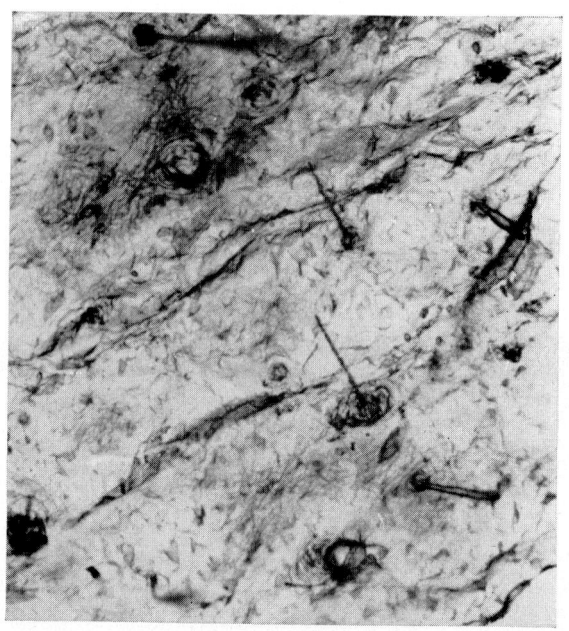

Fig. 3.—Skin surface biopsy from cheek to show numerous small follicle openings and inconspicuous skin markings. (Unstained; × 11.)

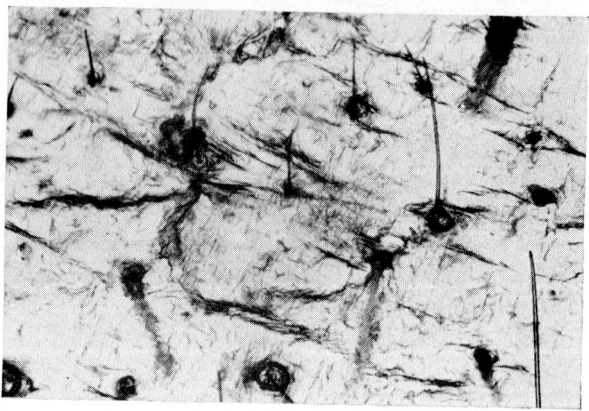

Fig. 4.—Skin surface biopsy from forehead. (Unstained; × 7·5).

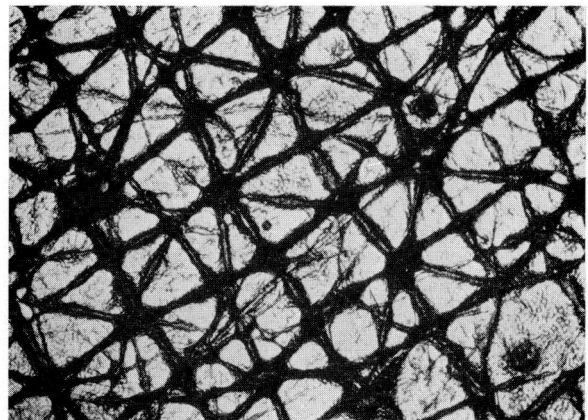

Fig. 5.—Skin surface biopsy from forearm. There is a rhomboidal pattern which constrasts strikingly with the less prominent and regular patterning on the face. (Unstained; × 7·5.)

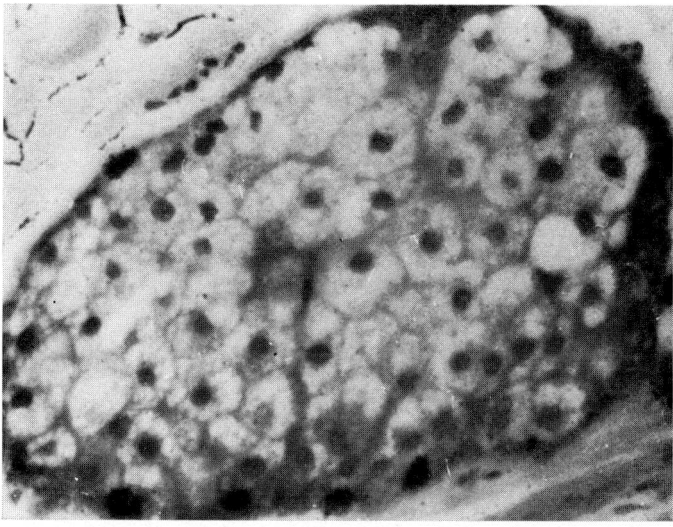

Fig. 6.—Autoradiograph of biopsy of facial skin to show sebaceous gland with 'labelled' cells in DNA synthesis at the periphery. (HE; × 300.)

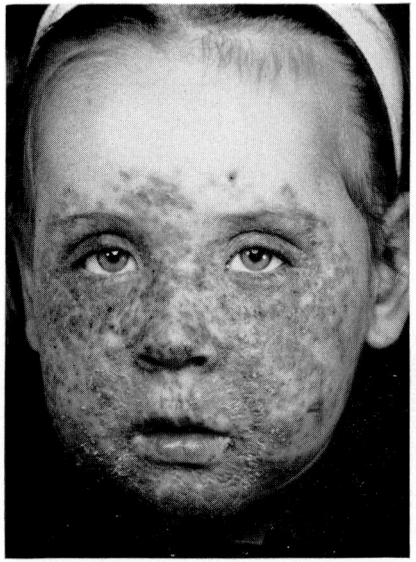

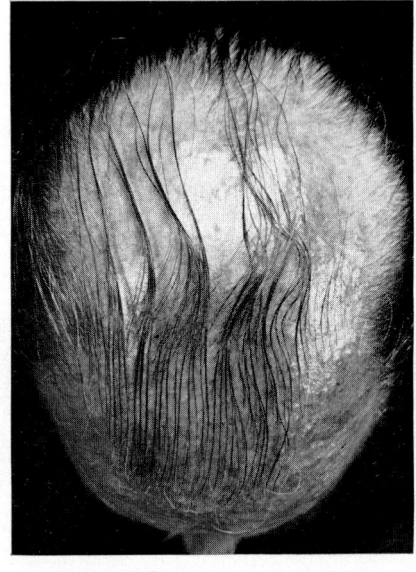

Fig. 7.—Rosacea-like disorder in child treated with steroids.

Fig. 9.—Rosacea in the 'bald patch'.

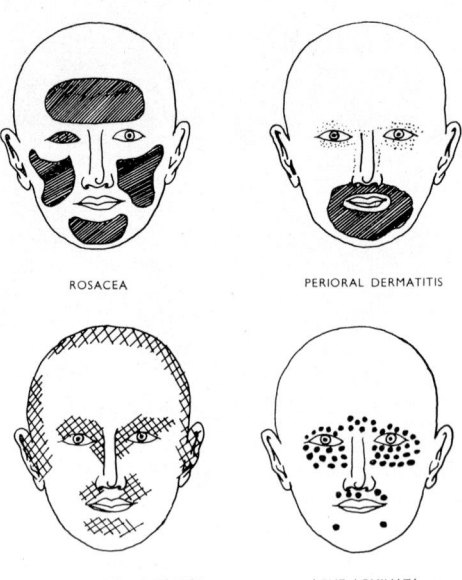

ROSACEA

PERIORAL DERMATITIS

SEBORRHOEIC DERMATITIS

ACNE AGMINATA

Fig. 8.—Diagram to show distribution of four facial rashes.

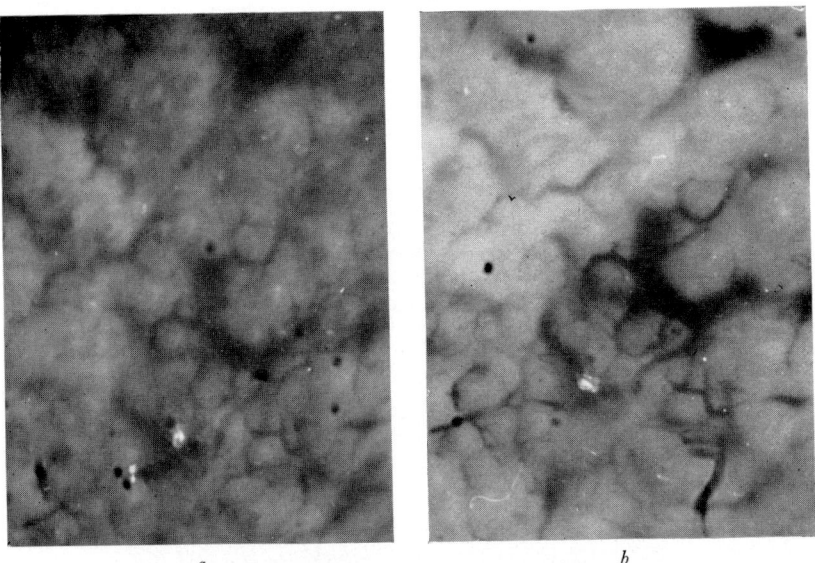

Fig. 10.—Capillary photomicrographs before (*a*) and after (*b*) exposure to 1 : 10 000 adrenaline solution.

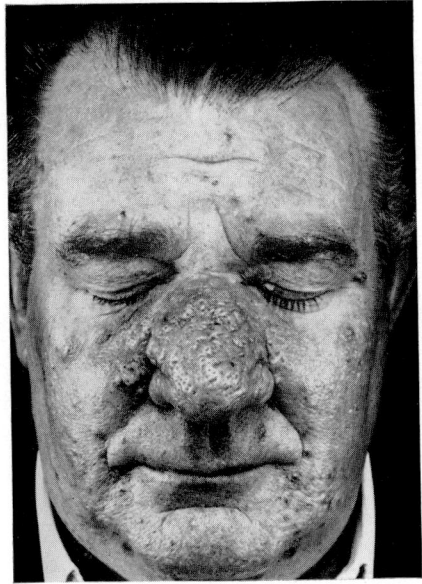

Fig. 11.—Rhinophyma showing irregular hypertrophy and prominence of pilosebaceous orifices.

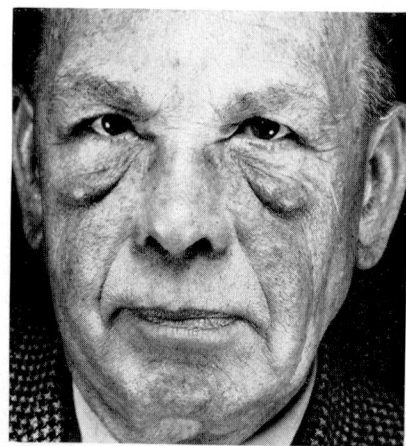

Fig. 12.—Facial lymphoedema in a man who has had mild rosacea.

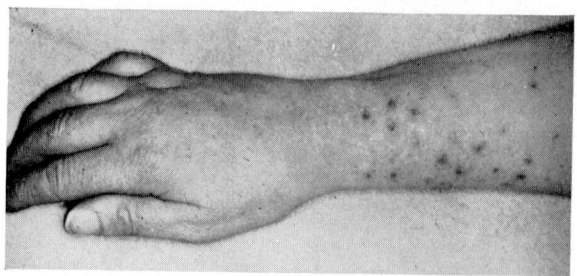

Fig. 13.—Papules on the arm in 'disseminated rosacea'.

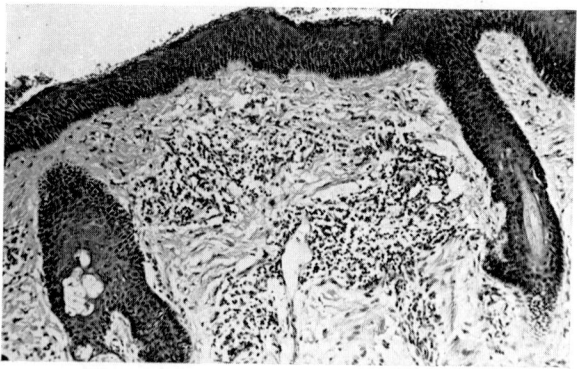

Fig. 14.—Histological section from patient with rosacea. The inflammatory infiltrate is distributed predominantly perivascularly. (HE; ×45.)

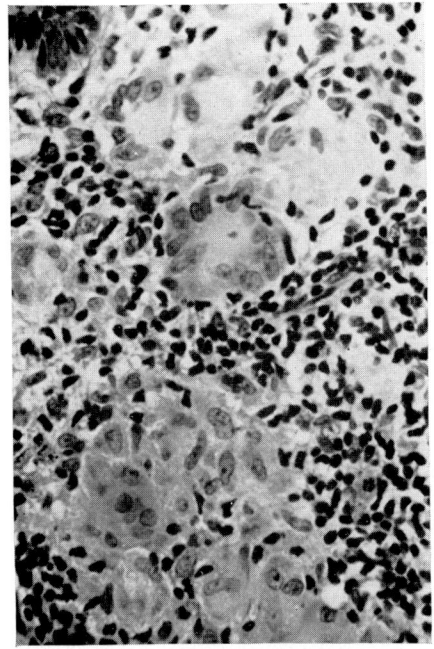

Fig. 15.—Granulomatous infiltrate in rosacea with many giant cells. (HE; × 175.)

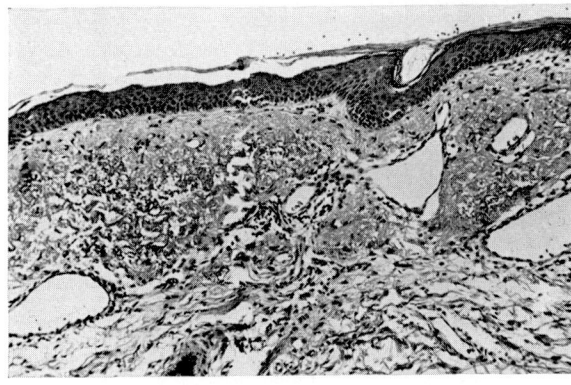

Fig. 16.—Solar elastotic change, oedema, telangiectasia and dermal disorganization in the upper dermis in a patient with rosacea. (HE; × 45.)

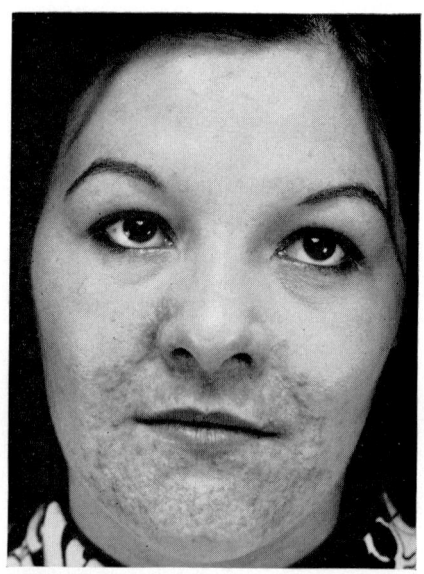

Fig. 17.—Perioral dermatitis. Typical distribution around mouth of rash composed of many small papules and pustules.

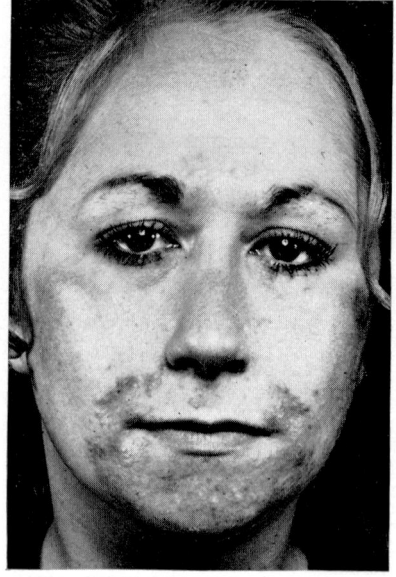

Fig. 18.—Another patient with typical perioral dermatitis. The perioral sparing is well shown here.

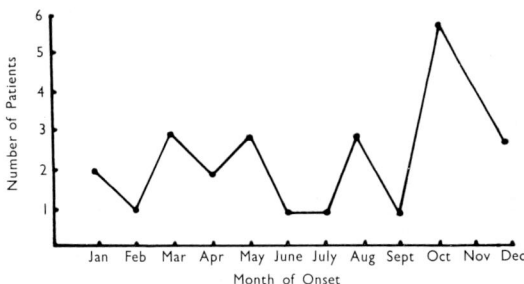

Fig. 19.—Diagram to show month of onset in new patients with perioral dermatitis in a recent study.

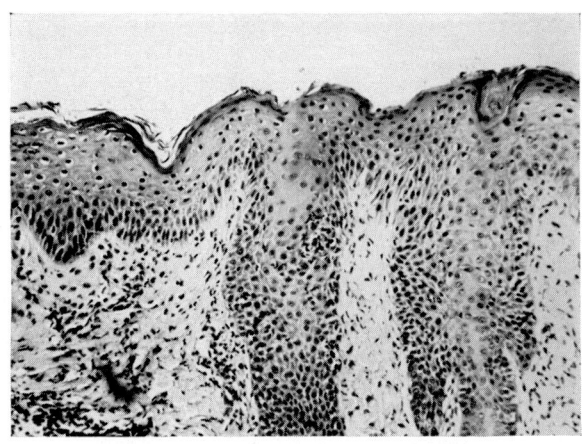

Fig. 20.—The histology of perioral dermatitis showing eczematous changes and inflammation in follicles. (HE; × 45.)

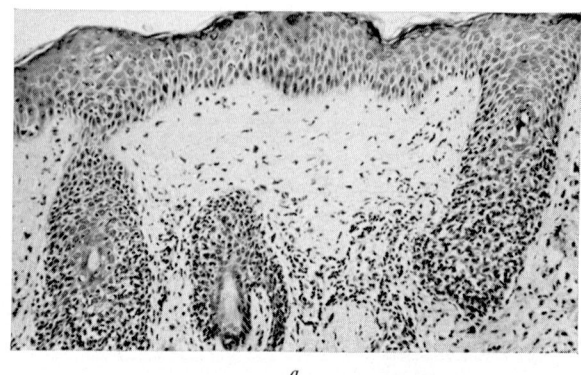

a

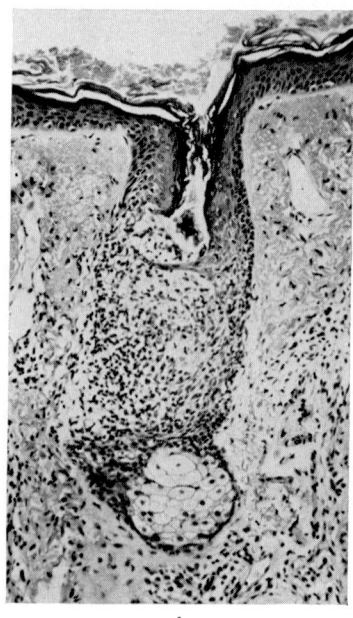

b

Fig. 21*a, b.*—Histology of perioral dermatitis showing spongiosis and inflammation of hair follicles. (HE; ×45.)

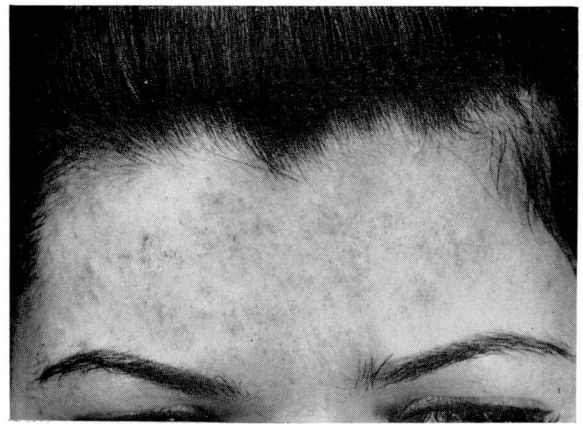

Fig. 22.—Patient with mild acne of the forehead showing many blackheads.

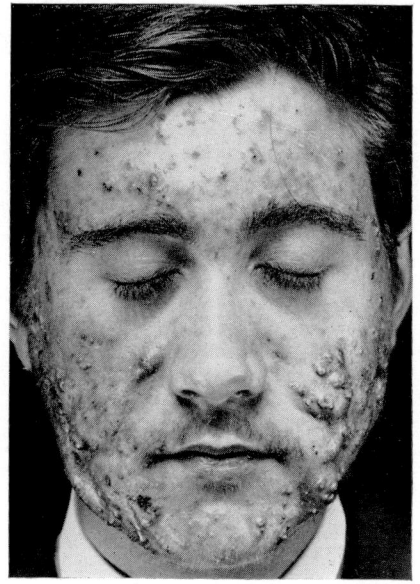

Fig. 23.—Severe cystic acne affecting the cheeks.

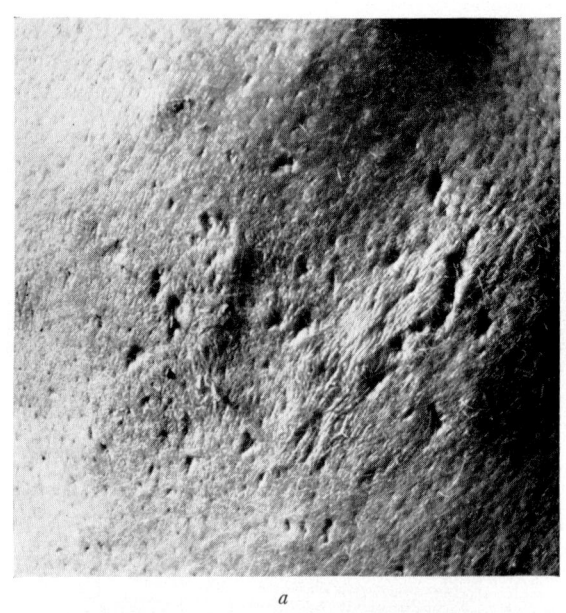

a

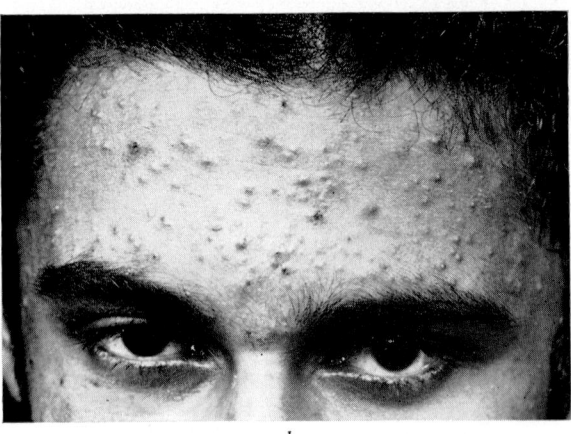

b

Fig. 24.—*a*, Shallow pock and pitted scars resulting from acne on the cheek. *b*, Papulopustular acne affecting the forehead.

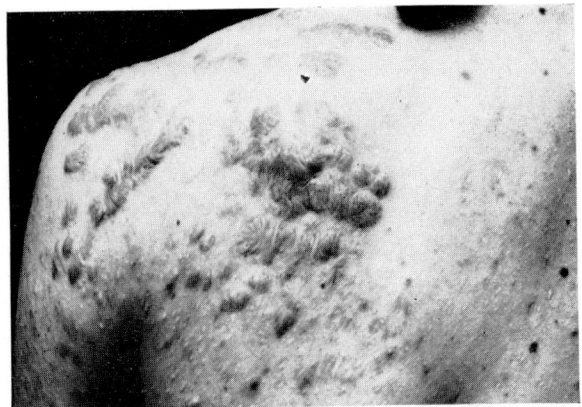

Fig. 25.—Keloid and hypertrophic scarring affecting the back as a result of cystic acne.

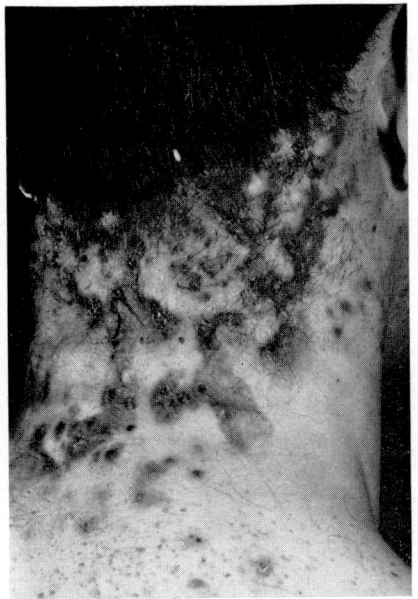

Fig. 26.—Severe cystic acne of the back of the neck with draining sinuses and hypertrophic scars.

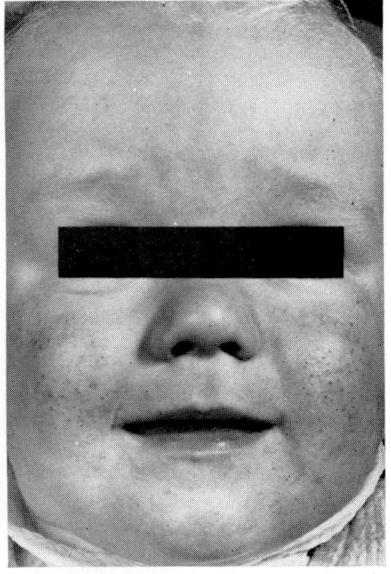

Fig. 27.—Mild acne affecting a child. There are many comedones and a few papules.

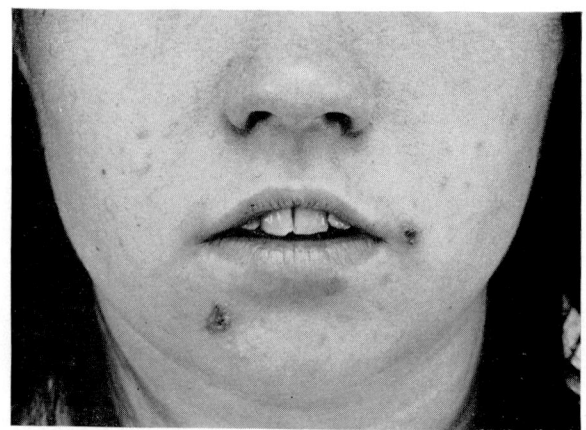

Fig. 28.—Excoriated acne (*'acné excoriée des jeunes filles'*).

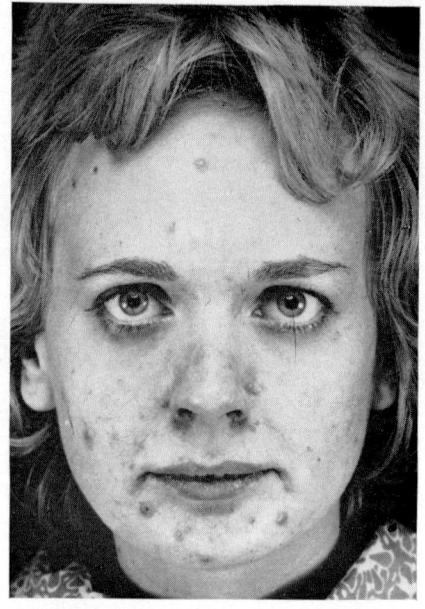

Fig. 29.—Papular acne in a woman. The chin is disproportionately affected. This type of acne often shows a premenstrual 'flare'.

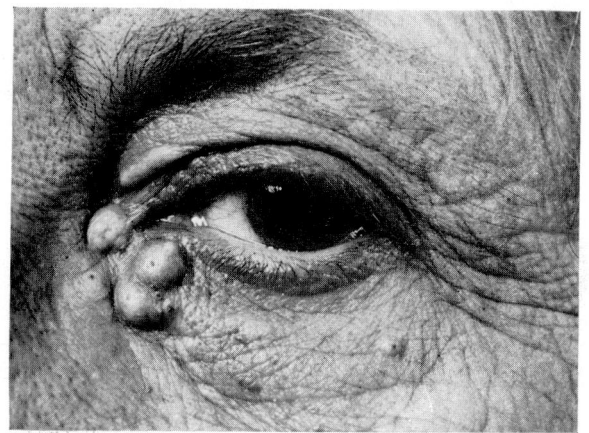

Fig. 30.—Senile comedones in a man aged 65.

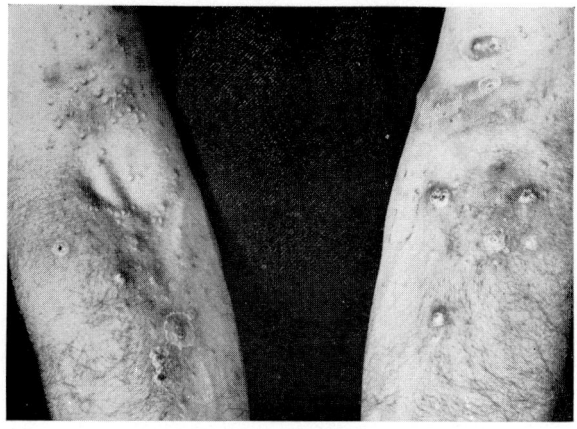

Fig. 31.—Cystic acne involving forearms in individual with chloracne.

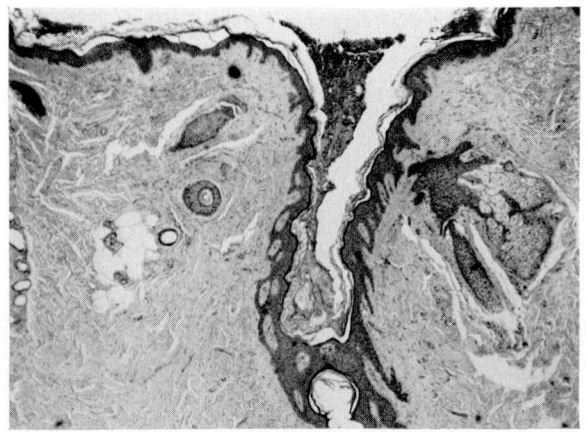

Fig. 32.—Dilated follicle showing irregular hypertrophy of follicle wall. (HE; × 15.)

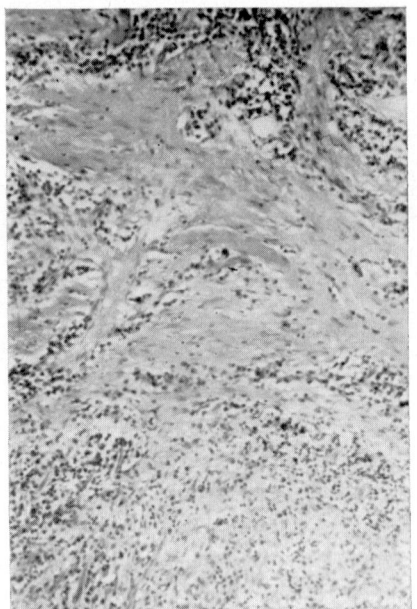

Fig. 33.—Section from sycosis nuchae showing fibrosis and plasma cells.

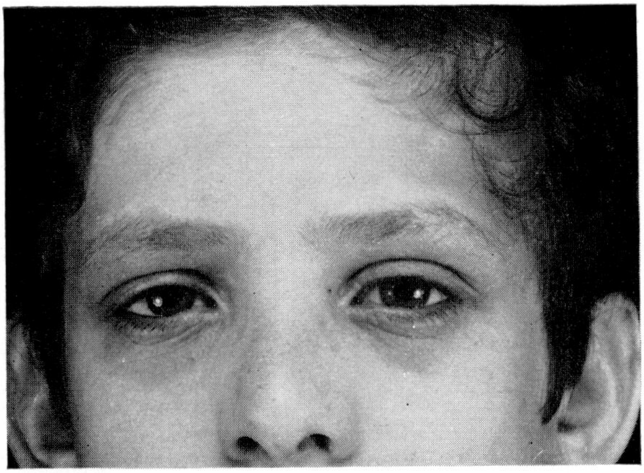

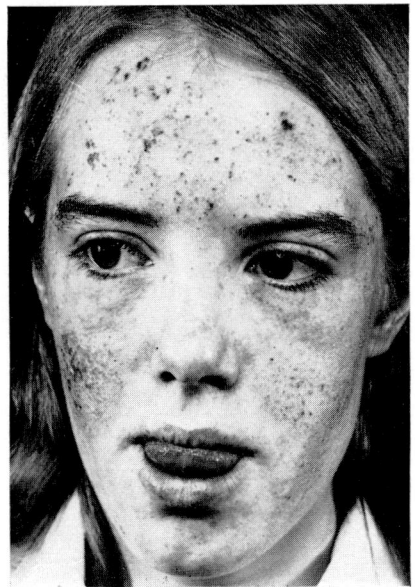

Fig. 34.—Atopic facies. There seems to be an extra skin crease around the eyes and there is comparative pallor on the cheeks.

Fig. 35.—Exudative atopic dermatitis affecting the face.

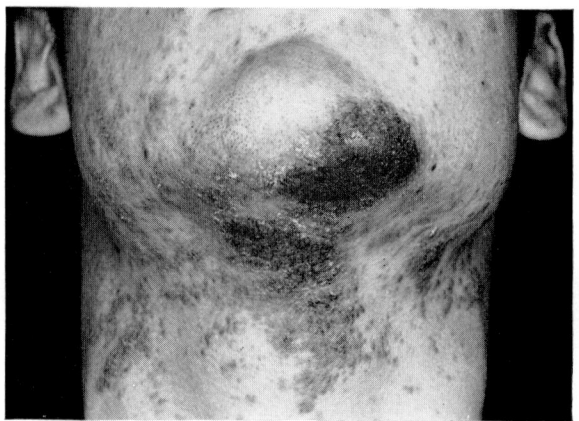

Fig. 36.—Crusted eczema with similarities to impetigo.

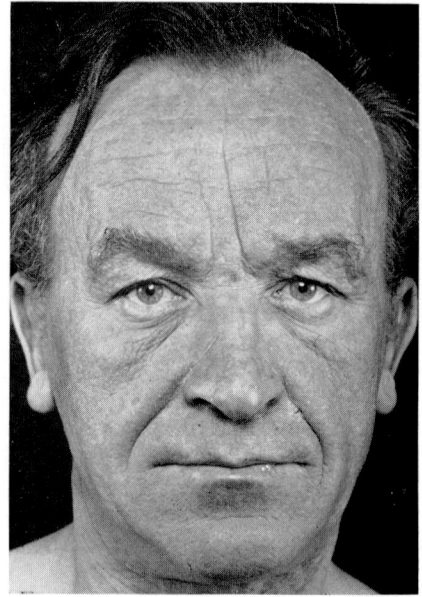

Fig. 37.—This man had an allergic contact dermatitis to a rubber additive (MBT).

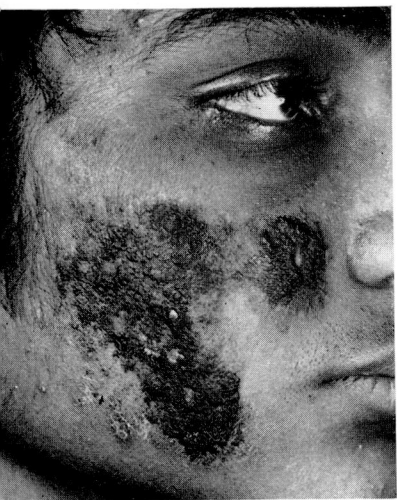

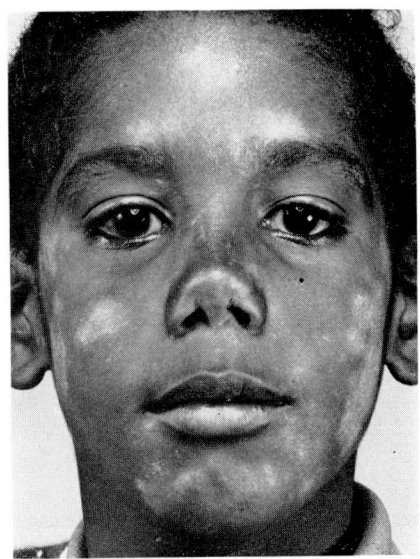

Fig. 38.—This young man developed a primary irritant dermatitis after starting topical treatment with a sulphur preparation for his acne.

Fig. 39.—Pityriasis simplex in a Negro child.

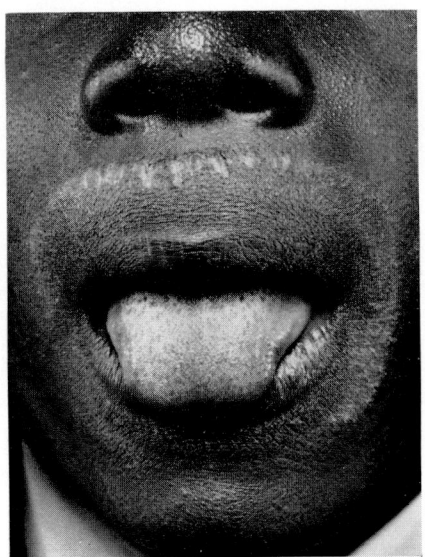

Fig. 40.—Lip-licking cheilitis. There is a circumoral area of dermatitis. This cleared when the child stopped the habit.

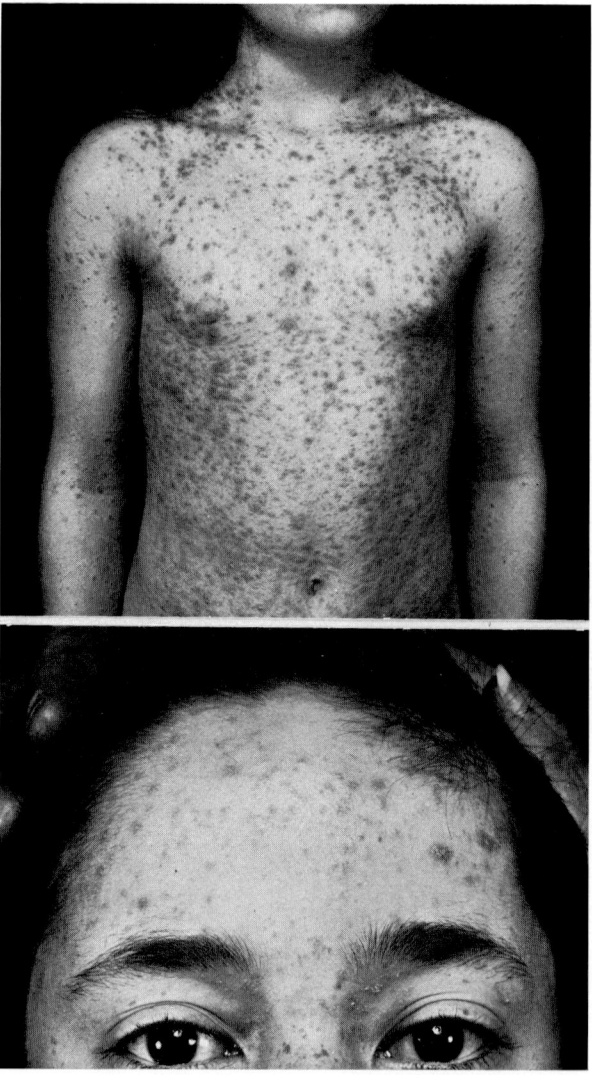

Fig. 41.—This child had typical pityriasis rosea with lesions of the forehead as well.

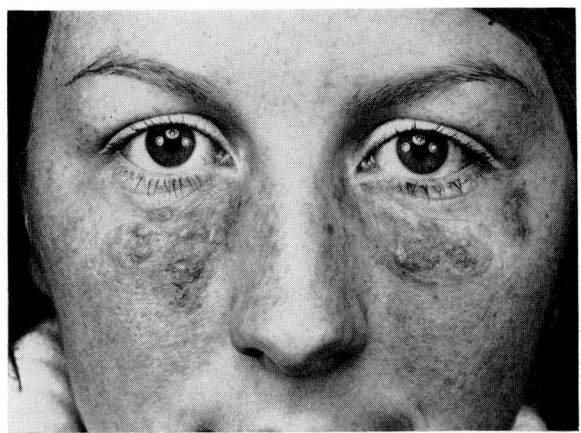

Fig. 42.—Facial lesions of discoid LE with adherent scales, telangiectasia and atrophy.

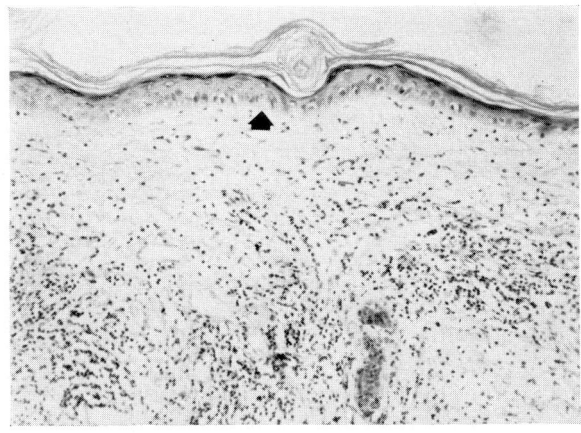

Fig. 43.—Histology of discoid LE. There is relative hyperkeratosis and slight epidermal thinning. In places the basal layer of the epidermis is damaged and there are a few homogenized eosinophilic cells scattered along its length (arrow). The upper dermis is oedematous and there are many lymphocytes perivascularly. (HE; × 45.)

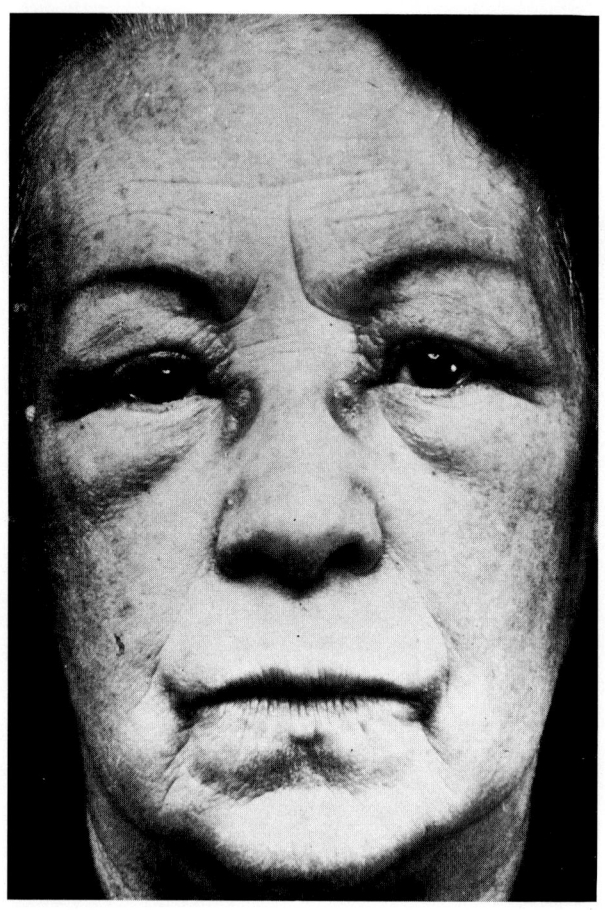

Fig. 44.—Acute dermatomyositis showing pronounced periorbital swelling.

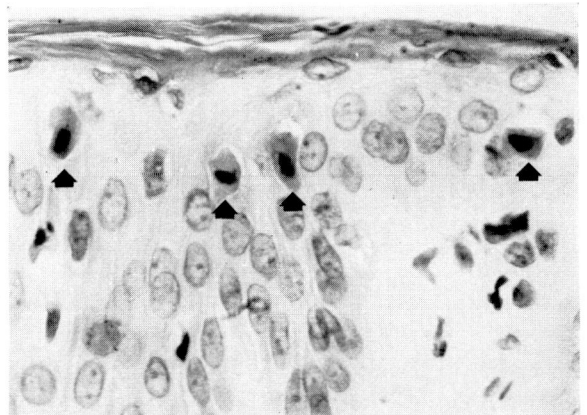

Fig. 45.—Scattered through the epidermis are eosinophilic cells with pyknotic nuclei—the so-called 'sunburn cells' (arrows). (HE; × 140.)

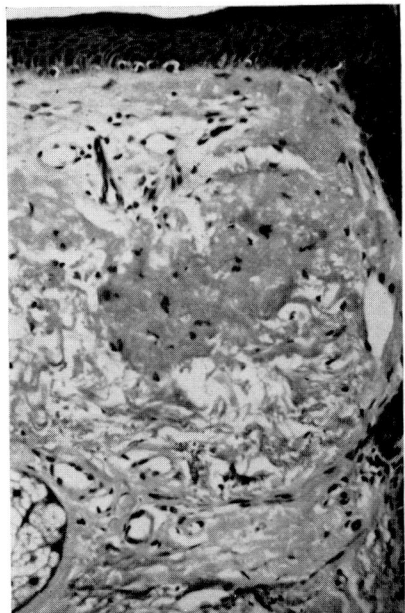

Fig. 46.—Marked solar elastosis in papillary and upper dermis. The affected tissue has lost its normal fibrillary structure and is homogenized and disorganized. (HE; × 45.)

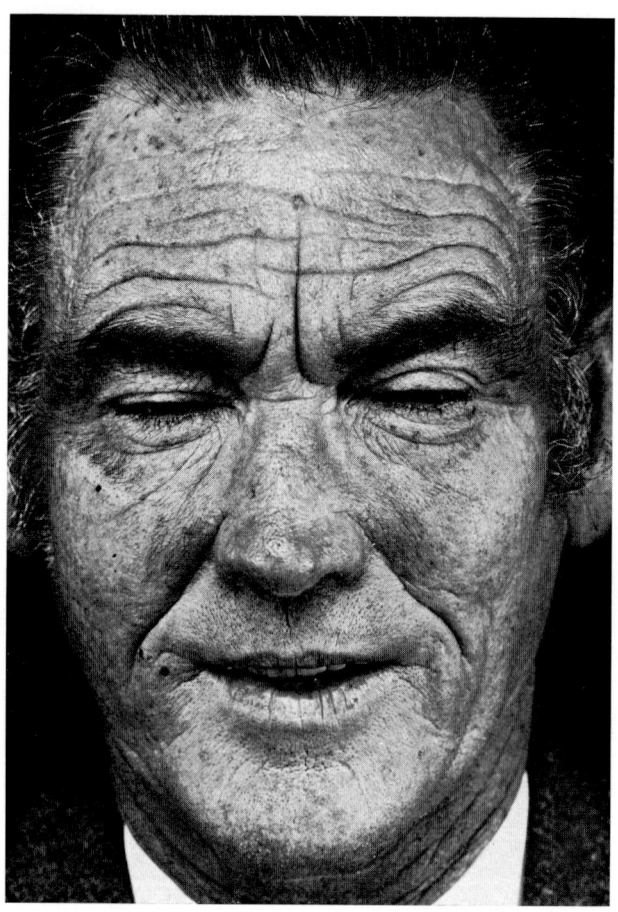

Fig. 47.—Man with porphyria cutanea tarda. Note the increase in terminal hair around the eyes and on the cheeks. Some erosions and skin thickening can also be seen.

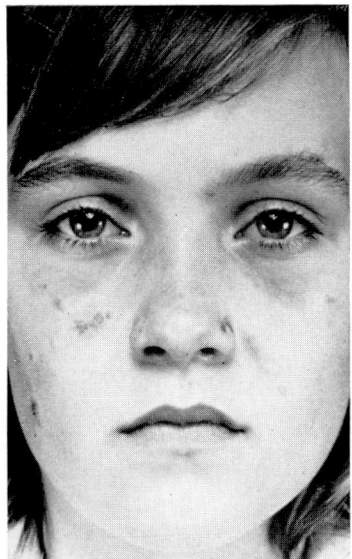

Fig. 48.—Hutchinson's summer prurigo in a young girl. There is an excoriated eczematous prurigo type of rash on the cheeks and nose.

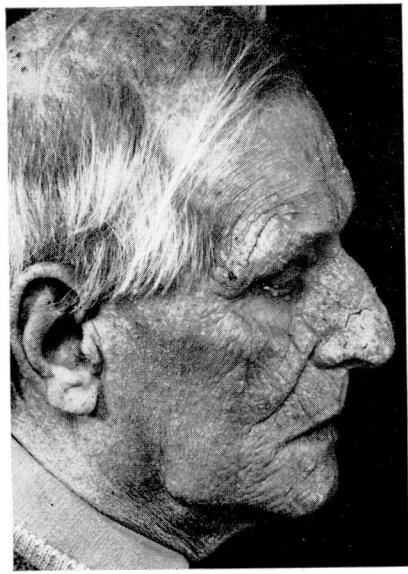

Fig. 49.—Actinic reticuloid showing severe eczematous change with lichenification and thickening of facial skin.

5

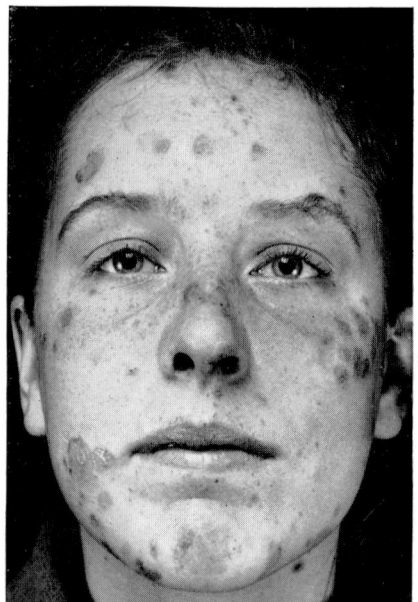

Fig. 50.—Typical impetigo.

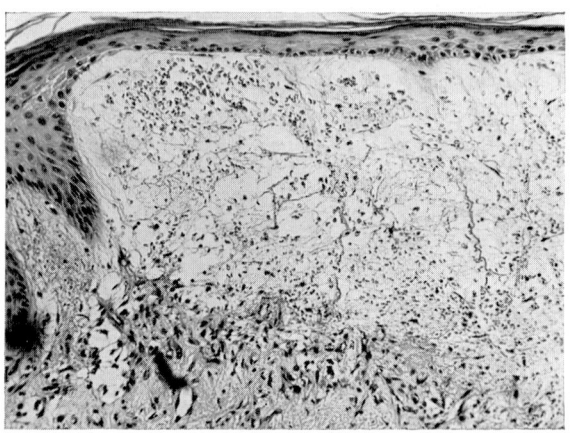

Fig. 51.—Histopathology of erysipelas showing a subepidermal area of intense oedema and haemorrhage. (HE; ×45.)

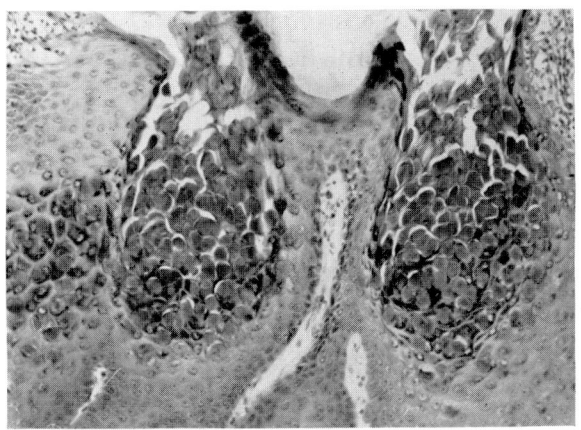

Fig. 52.—Histopathology of molluscum contagiosum showing characteristic degeneration of epidermal cells with globular molluscum bodies. (HE; ×60.)

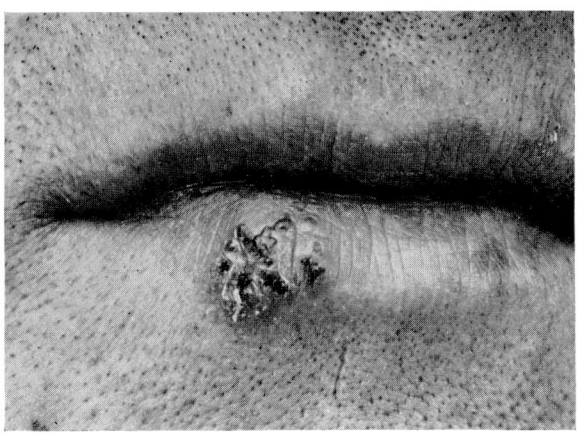

Fig. 53.—Typical herpes simplex lesion of lip.

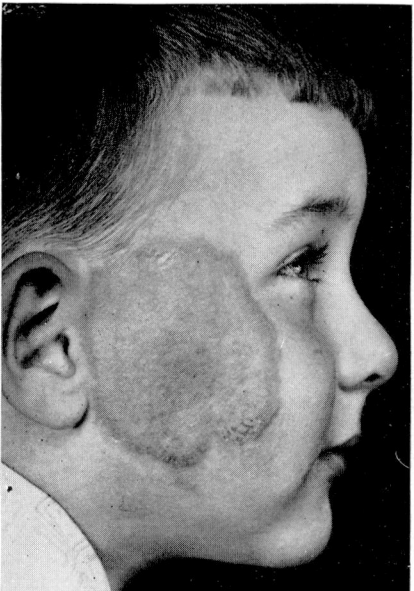

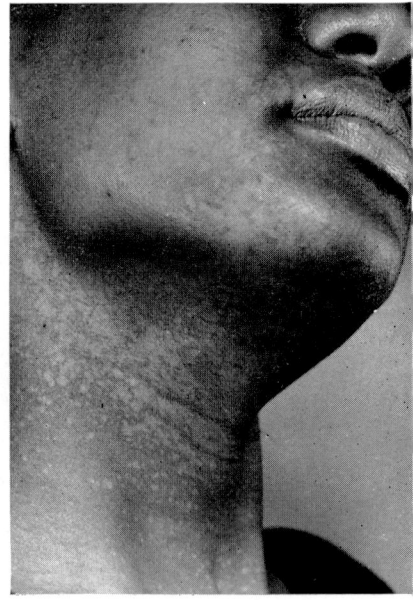

Fig. 54.—Ringworm of the face.

Fig. 56.—Pityriasis versicolor affecting the neck and face.

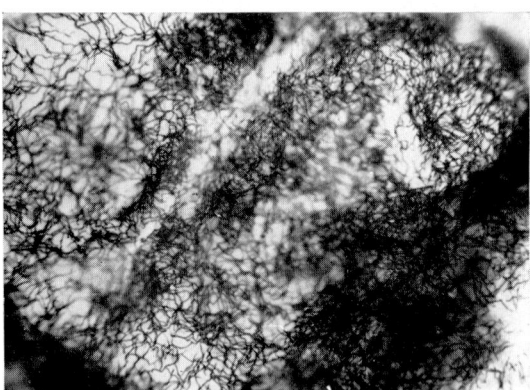

Fig. 55.—Skin surface biopsy stained by periodic acid–Schiff method to show large amounts of ringworm fungus.

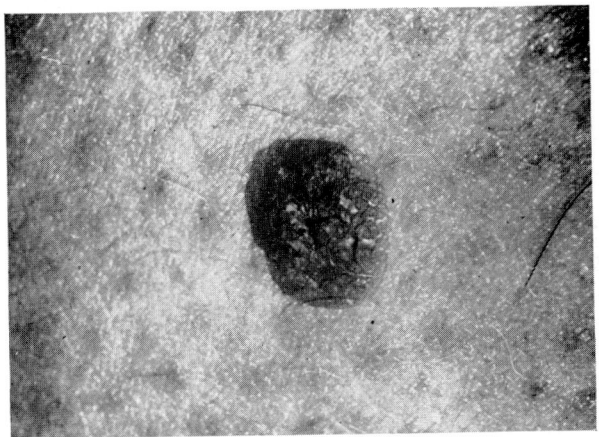

Fig. 57.—Close view of seborrhoeic wart on the face of elderly lady. It is lobulated, pigmented and slightly scaly.

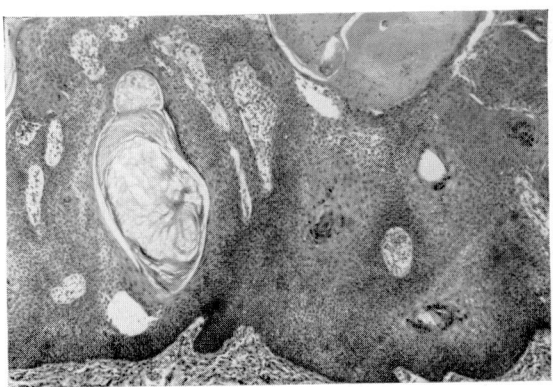

Fig. 58.—Histopathology of seborrhoeic wart showing immature keratinocytes, apparent 'dermal islands', areas of keratinization and degeneration. (HE; ×22.)

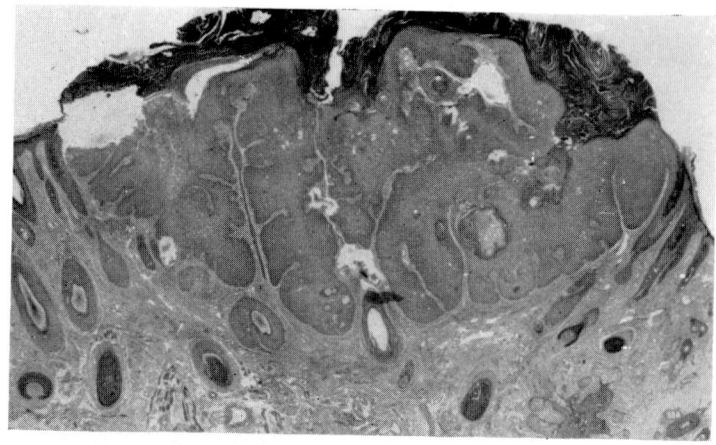

a

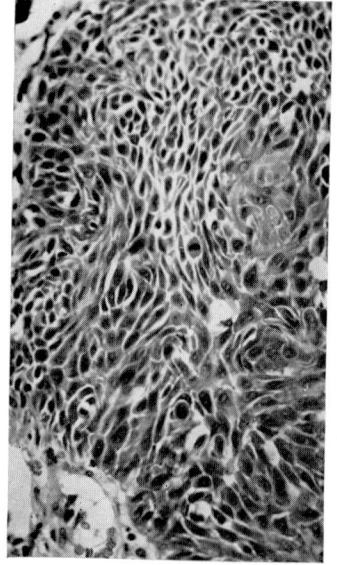

b

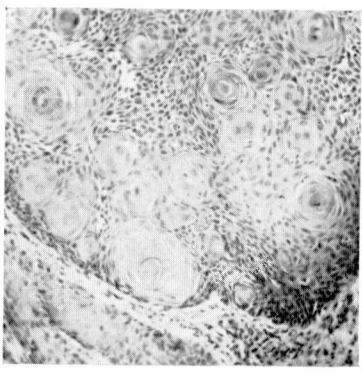

c

Fig. 59.—Histopathology of inverted follicular keratosis. *a,* Low power view of an inverted follicular keratosis showing a 'partially' inverted architecture. (HE; × 5·4.) *b,* Detail of similar lesion showing many mitotic figures—also a feature of an irritated seborrhoeic wart. (HE; × 120.) *c,* Detail of similar lesion showing 'squamoid eddies'— also a feature of an irritated seborrhoeic wart. (HE; × 45.)

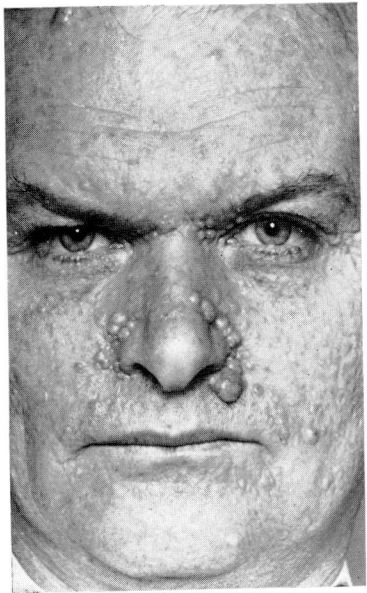

Fig. 60.—Typical multiple lesions of tricho-epithelioma.

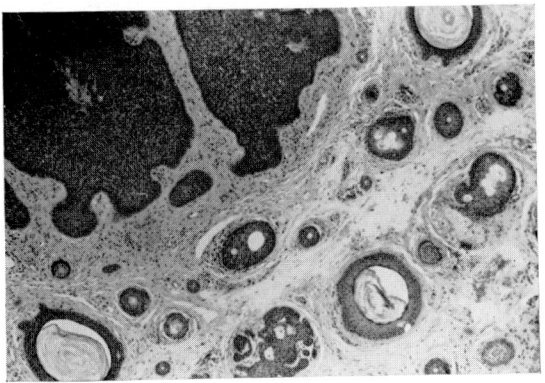

Fig. 61.—Histopathology of tricho-epithelioma.

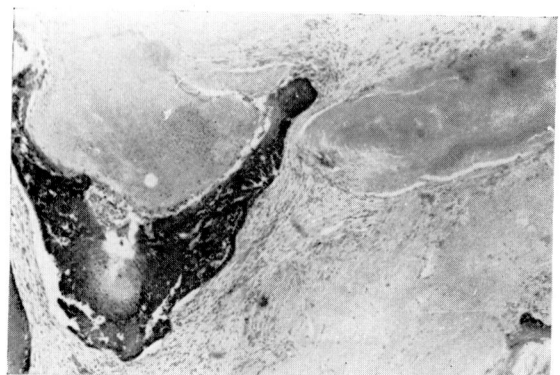

Fig. 62.—Histopathology of pilomatrixoma.

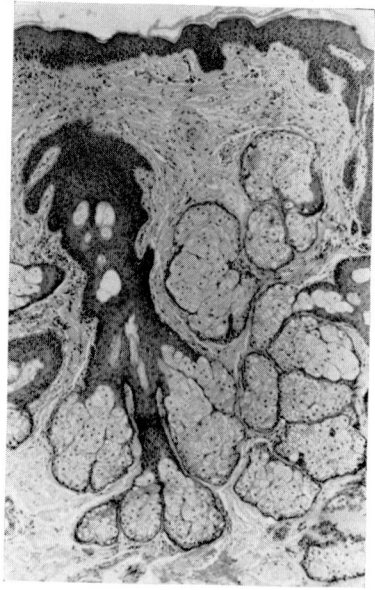

Fig. 63.—Histopathology of senile sebaceous gland hypertrophy.

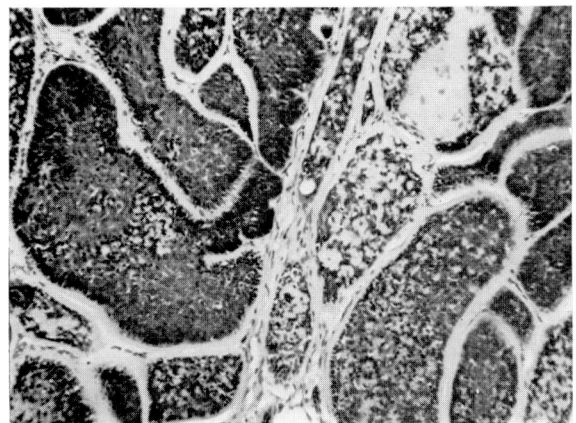

Fig. 64.—Histopathology of cylindroma of the scalp.

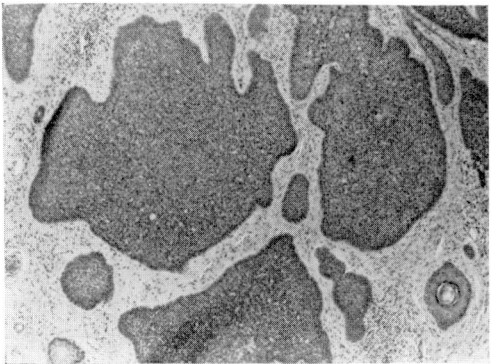

Fig. 65.—Histopathology of basal cell carcinoma.

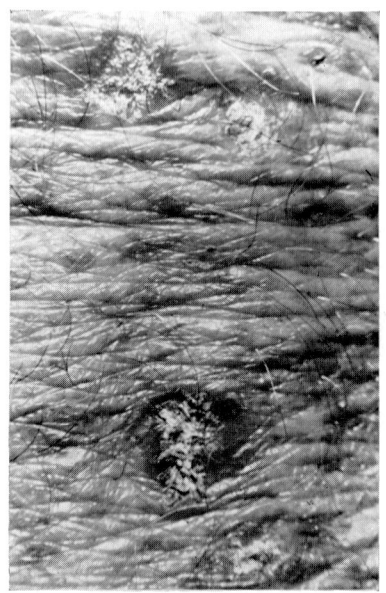

Fig. 66.—Close view of solar keratoses.

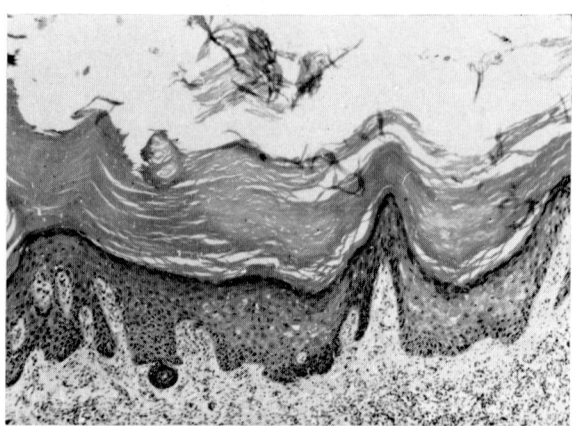

Fig. 67.—Histopathology of solar keratosis showing large cells with abnormal nuclei at base of epidermis. (HE; ×22.)

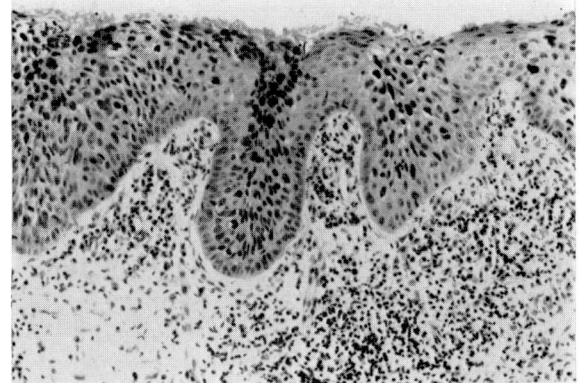

Fig. 68.—Histopathology of Bowen's disease showing cells with abnormal large hyperchromatic nuclei throughout epidermis. (HE; ×90.)

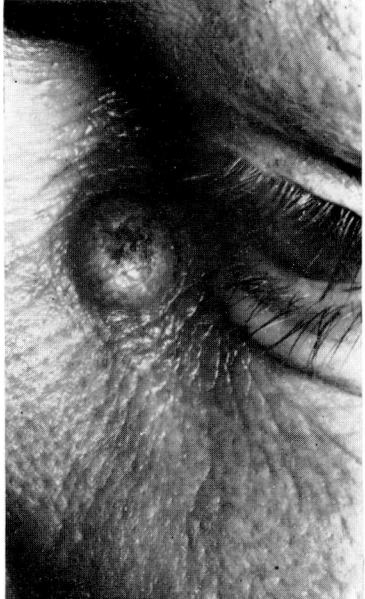

Fig. 69.—Typical kerato-acanthoma with a central plug.

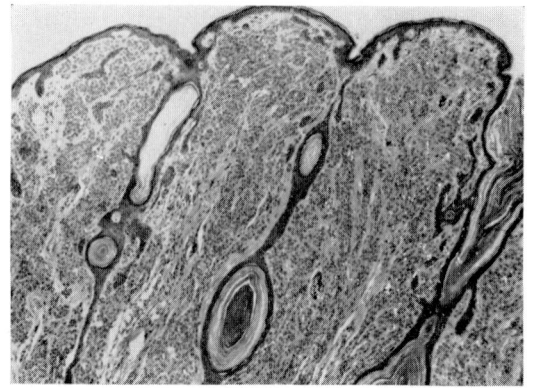

Fig. 70.—Histopathology of a dermal cellular naevus showing numerous aggregates of typical naevus cells. (HE; × 15.)

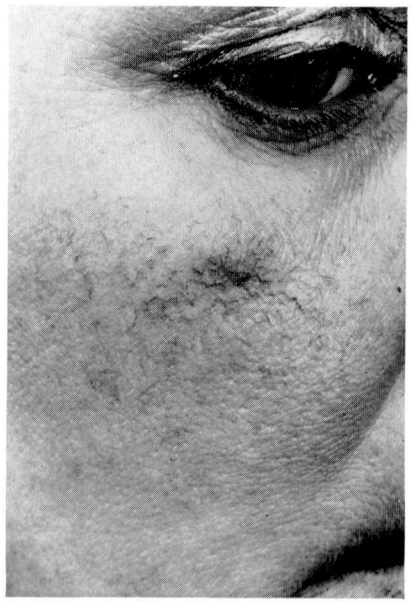

Fig. 71.—Spider naevus on cheek.

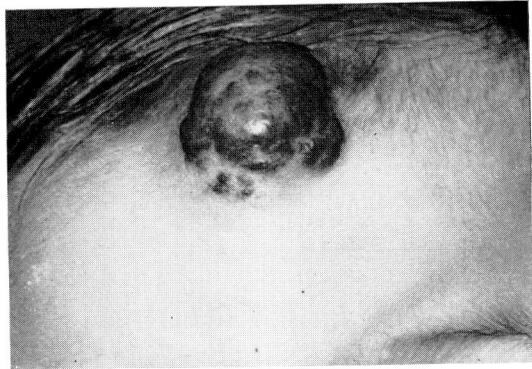

Fig. 72.—Large capillary haemangioma ('strawberry naevus') on forehead of infant.

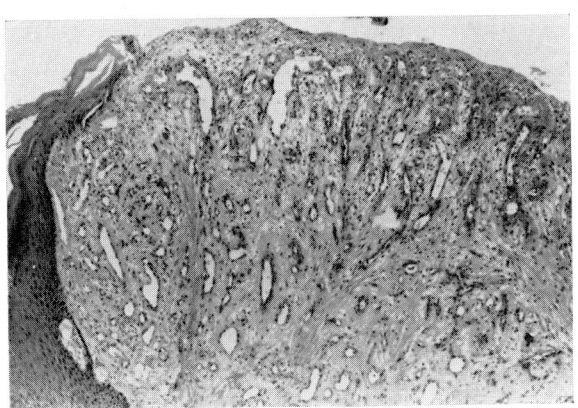

Fig. 73.—Histopathology of pyogenic granuloma.

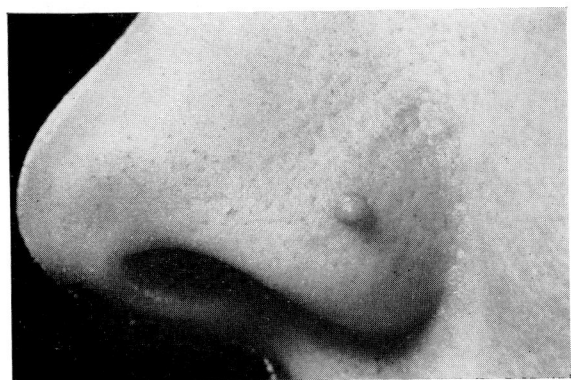

Fig. 74.—Fibrous papule of the nose.

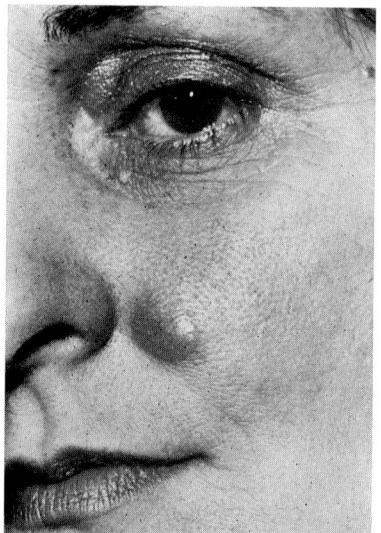

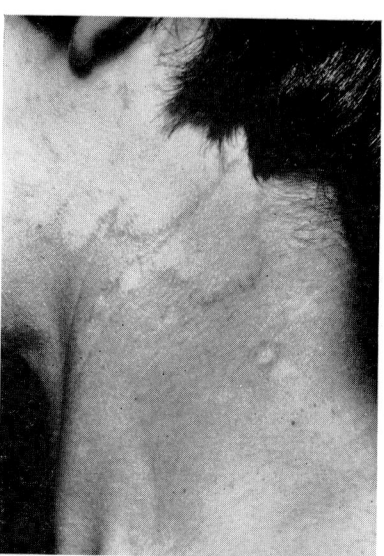

Fig. 75.—Lesion of granuloma faciale.

Fig. 76.—Facial necrobiosis lipoidica.

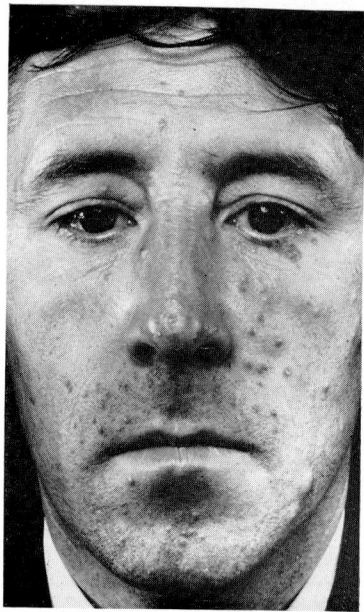

Fig. 77.—Acne agminata. There are many dark-red and brownish papules on the lower cheeks, nose, chin, forehead and around the eyes.

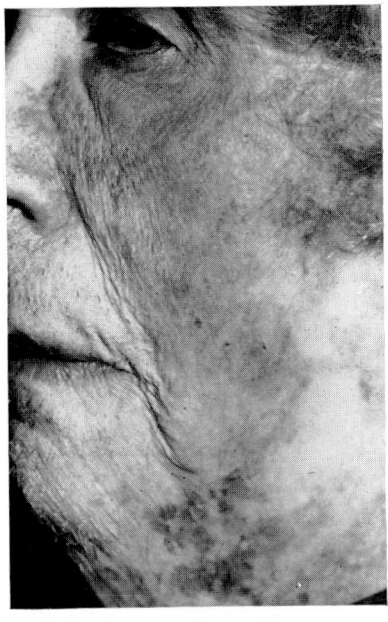

a

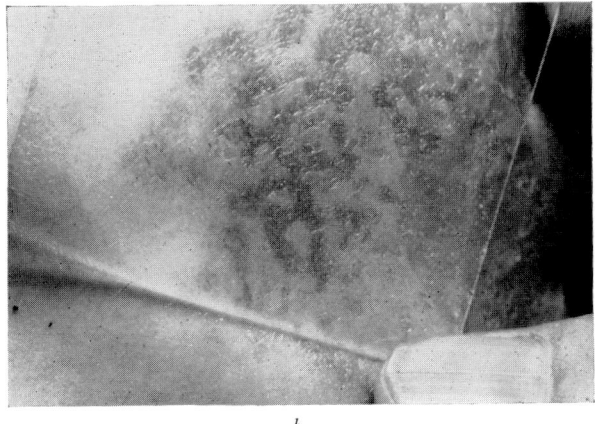

b

Fig. 78.—*a*, Lupus vulgaris in elderly lady with severe scarring. *b*, Diascopy of area of lupus vulgaris showing 'apple jelly nodules'.

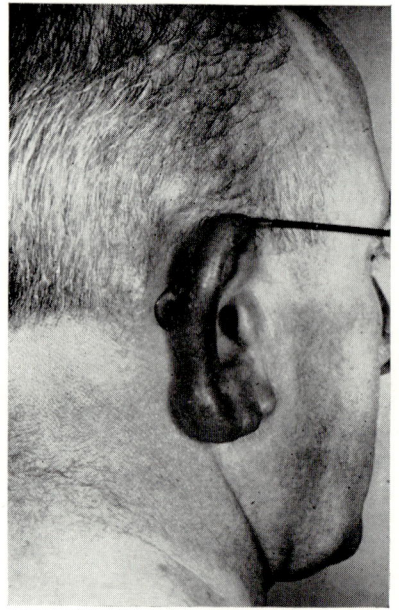

Fig. 79.—Lupus pernio affecting the ear.

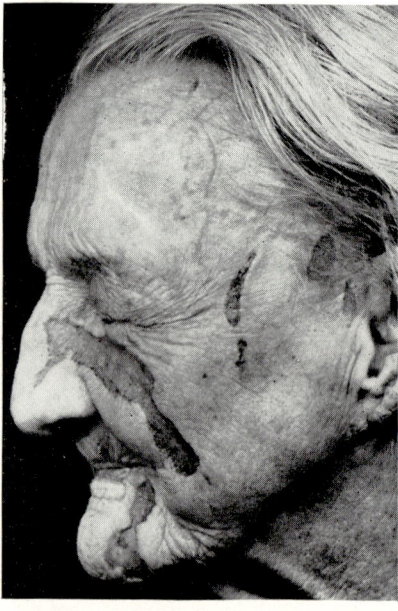

Fig. 81.—Artefactual lesions on the face of elderly lady who had a lesion of the trigeminal ganglion.

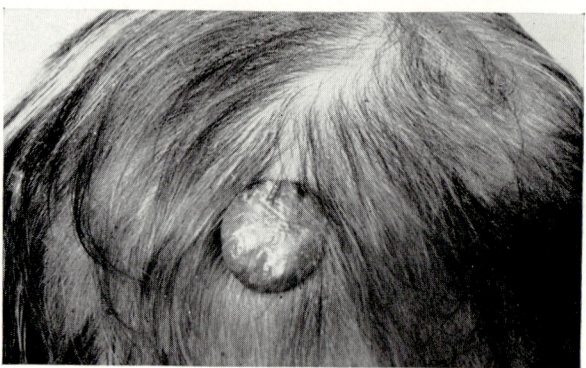

Fig. 80.—Juvenile xanthogranuloma on scalp. This lesion was orange-yellow and there were several others scattered on the body.

Chapter 1

Anatomy, Physiology, Microbiology and Special Pathology

Facial skin possesses certain special characteristics which it is helpful to understand in order to obtain a dynamic view of facial dermatoses. It should also be appreciated that there are regional differences on the skin of the face itself, and these are also important in influencing the pattern of diseases of facial skin.

EPIDERMAL STRUCTURES

From *Fig.* 1 it can be seen that the usual markedly wavy outline to the basal layer of the epidermis seen on most other body sites has given way to more gentle undulations. This loss of the epidermal rete pattern (and at the same time the dermal papilla) is of fundamental importance, as will become evident later. The loss of rete pattern and of the papillae is more obvious over the cheeks, and to a lesser extent on the forehead and chin.

In addition, the epidermis is thinner than that on many parts of the body or limbs. The number of cells constituting the depth of the epidermis is, perhaps, one or two cells less than on the epidermis of the trunk and limbs. It is easy to misdiagnose epidermal atrophy when presented with a section of normal facial skin. The granular layer is particularly difficult to find and the stratum corneum is thinner than in most other parts of the body.

The horny layer is almost absent on the eyelids. The stratum corneum of the 'beard area', of the forehead and of the cheek have distinct patterns when examined by skin surface biopsy (Marks and Dawber, 1971) (*Figs.* 2, 3, 4, 5). In this technique the stratum corneum is stripped off in one coherent layer using a rapidly bonding cyano-acrylate adhesive; this method has many applications and will be mentioned again later. It is noticeable that the usual rhomboidal or diamond patterning of the stratum corneum is absent from facial skin. It can be seen that there is a distinctive perifollicular horny ring that is particularly well marked in the sample from the beard area.

I

The significance of this patterning of the stratum corneum is unknown; the absence of the rhomboidal pattern seen in most other sites might be related to the loss of the epidermal ridge and papilla pattern.

HAIR FOLLICLES AND SEBACEOUS GLANDS

The face is particularly well supplied with hair follicles and sebaceous glands. It has been estimated that there are 850 per sq cm on the forehead compared to 50–100 per sq cm on the back of the hand.

Although the term 'sebaceous follicles' is frequently used for the follicular structures over the nose and the cheeks, serial sectioning will usually reveal a hair structure of some kind even if it is only very small. Many of the follicles in the acne areas possess more than one opening and are known as 'polyostotic'.

The Sebaceous Glands

These are holocrine glands and mature sebaceous gland cells are formed by a process of differentiation that begins shortly after the cells are formed at the periphery of the gland. The peripheral cells divide more frequently than the germinative cells of the interfollicular epidermis (Epstein and Epstein, 1966). The high labelling index demonstrated autoradiographically after the intracutaneous injection of tritiated thymidine is seen in *Fig.* 6. The rate of secretion of sebum is ultimately dependent on the rate of sebaceous cell formation and this is under hormonal control—predominantly androgenic. Thus the anatomical sites where the density and size of the sebaceous glands are greatest will show the greatest rate of sebaceous secretion. These correspond fairly well to the acne-prone areas, i.e. the forehead, chin, cheeks, front of chest and upper back. Occasionally sebaceous glands are found in the lips and are visible as rows of yellowish-white blobs. This normal finding is sometimes known as Fordyce's disease.

SWEAT GLANDS

Eccrine sweat secretory coils and ducts are abundant on the face. Eccrine sweat secretion depends on both thermal and emotional stimuli. The forehead, in particular, sweats in response to emotional as well as thermal stimuli. Occasionally, because of an aberrant nerve supply, 'gustatory' stimuli induce sweating (Watkins, 1973). 'Gustatory sweating' in response to spices or other pungent foods may be seen all over the face, but is well marked over the forehead and cheeks. Apocrine sweat glands are usually confined to the scalp but may occasionally be seen on the forehead. They appear to have no special function in this situation.

NERVES

The face, as might be expected from the extreme sensitivity of the facial skin, is extremely well supplied with cutaneous nerves. Montagna et al. (1964) found in a histochemical investigation that the face had more cholinesterase-containing nerves than anywhere in the body apart from the external genitalia. In addition, the complex inter-twinings of nerve networks around the pilary canal that constitute the 'hair end-organ', were found by the same authors to be more numerous and better differentiated in facial skin. The chin and the jowl were found to be particularly well supplied, and apparently, in these areas, superficial nerve plexuses were formed at the junction of the pilary canal and the surface epidermis, from which occasional twigs rose up to the epidermis and seemed to penetrate it. In some areas of the facial skin the eccrine sweat ducts were also surrounded by a dense network of interwoven nerves. The sensory innervation to the face is supplied by the divisions of the fifth nerve.

The skin of the lower jaw anterior to the pre-auricular region is innervated by the mandibular division after it has traversed the mandibular canal in the mandible. The cheek, upper lip and lower eyelid are supplied by branches of the maxillary branch of the fifth after it emerges from the foramen rotundum. The ophthalmic branch of the fifth nerve supplies the conjunctiva, the upper eyelid, most of the nose, the forehead and part of the scalp. The greater, lesser and third auricular nerves, which are branches of the cervical plexus, supply part of the skin of the neck and the external ear.

BLOOD SUPPLY TO THE FACE

The external carotid artery supplies blood to the facial skin via the facial and superficial temporal arteries. Pinkness of the cheeks is due to visibility of the subpapillary venous plexus and although cosmetically desirable is not necessarily indicative of health. The ease with which this plexus can be seen is a reflection of the loss of the 'ridge and papilla' pattern of the cheek epidermis with the consequence of shortening and even loss of the papillary capillaries. This arrangement of the small blood vessels of the facial skin explains the frequency with which telangiectasia appears in this site. It is often assumed that blood flow through facial skin is especially rapid because of the pinkness of this area. However, this is not necessarily so, as distension of the subpapillary venous plexus and a sluggish capillary blood flow can produce the same colour effect. Borrie (1955) found that there was no significant increase in skin surface temperature on the cheeks of rosacea patients despite the increase in redness.

Blushing

Comparatively little is known of the vasomotor controlling mechanisms for the skin of the face. It appears that the head and neck do not undergo as much vasoconstriction in response to cooling as the rest of the body.

Froese and Burton (1957) found that the heat loss from the head may amount to half the total resting heat production at -4 °C. Fox et al. (1962) investigated the vasomotor control of the skin of the head, neck and upper chest using thermometry with the 'heat transfer disc'. The nose, the lips and the ears were found to be predominantly controlled by vasoconstrictor impulses, and vasodilatation was due to release of vasoconstrictor tone. The blood supply of the cheeks, chin and forehead was different in that active vasodilatation took place as well as release of vasoconstrictor tone. It was suggested that the active vasodilatation was in some way connected with sweat gland activity. The flushing seen in the 'dumping syndrome' and in the carcinoid syndrome is due to increased blood levels of bradykinin rather than histamine or 5-hydroxytryptamine. It is not known whether blushing due to emotion, or the flushing seen with alcohol and other gastro-intestinal stimuli, or the 'hot flushes' of the menopause are due to the same or similar mechanisms. Recently it has been shown that clonidine significantly reduces the number of 'hot flushes' experienced at the menopause and it has been suggested that this is due to dampened reactivity of vessels of the facial skin (Clayden et al., 1974). It is obvious that the appearance of flushing depends on a number of factors besides the release of vasoconstrictor tone, the production of a vasodilatatory material or the opening up of shunts between plexuses at different anatomical levels. Flushing is difficult to see in a Negro (although it certainly occurs) because the heavily pigmented skin obscures it. Identification of a 'flush' will also depend on the degree of background erythema that already exists on the face. Presumably the ease with which a flush appears and its 'depth' depend to an extent on the distensibility of the small vessels of the subpapillary venous plexus. It is this last factor that seems to be of overriding importance in rosacea.

LYMPHATIC DRAINAGE

The face is one of the more common sites to find persistent lymphoedema and the lymph drainage seems only just adequate normally. Ellis et al. (1970) found that human serum albumin labelled with $^{131}I_2$ when injected intracutaneously into the normal cheek cleared more slowly than from other sites tested. Lymphatic pathways encircle the mouth and secondary deposits from carcinoma of the upper lip may be found in the submental glands (Larson et al., 1967). Generally the lymphatic drainage of the face is to the submental, submaxillary or parotid lymph nodes and thence to the anterior cervical chain of nodes.

THE DERMIS

The dermis is less thick and the connective tissue that it contains less dense and more loosely textured than that of most other sites on the body. This appearance is at least partially artefactual because of the abundance of adnexae. It also results from exposure to various climatic traumata including the sun (*see* Chapter 7). There is less subcutaneous fat in this region than in other sites. The muscles of facial expression are inserted into the lower parts of the dermis and occasionally muscle fragments are seen in biopsy specimens from these areas.

BIOPSY

Regrettably practitioners in the past have been content to issue advice and treatment without the intellectual exercise of making a diagnosis. Biopsy of facial lesions and rashes is often necessary for diagnosis and an understanding of the processes involved in many conditions. This procedure should not result in appreciable scar formation if simple precautions are taken as the facial skin heals particularly well after injury. The following are guidelines which the author has found helpful when performing biopsies of the face:
1. Wherever possible incisions should be parallel with the natural creases of the face. It is often helpful to ask the patient to smile and grimace when planning an incision.
2. Make the size of the biopsy as small as is compatible with providing enough tissue for a diagnosis.
3. The sharpest implements should be used (either scalpel or punch).
4. When suturing the wound margins, accurately oppose the margins; avoid tension at all costs and use fine silk sutures. Remove the sutures after 4 or 5 days.

Interpretation of Facial Biopsies
There are a few general points that are worth making with regard to the interpretation of biopsies from the skin of the face.
1. The epidermis and stratum corneum are thinner than in most other areas of the body. In addition the usual rete pattern is almost entirely absent. Consequently a mistaken impression of atrophy is sometimes obtained.
2. The dermis often shows the changes of solar elastosis. The intensity of this change depends on the history of solar exposure of

the individual and the degree of pigmentation (*see* Chapter 7). Individuals with rosacea and lupus erythematosus may be especially prone to this change.

3. The dermis is less compact and the superficial dermal blood vessels more dilated than in other areas. This may also be mistaken for atrophy.

4. The hair follicles and sebaceous glands are larger and more numerous than in all other sites apart from the scalp (the face has larger sebaceous glands than the scalp). This should be taken into account when assessing the presence of hypertrophy or hamartomata of these structures.

MICROBIOLOGY

The mite, *Demodex folliculorum*, is a frequently found commensal in biopsies from adult facial skin. In rosacea it has been suggested that *Demodex* plays a pathogenic role, but the evidence for this is slender (*see* Chapter 2). It lives in the pilary canal and never seems to penetrate the epidermis. The yeast-like micro-organism *Pityrosporon ovale* can also be found in or near the normal hair follicle. It frequently shows up as a collection of round or oval bodies in sections stained by the periodic acid–Schiff reagent.

The normal bacterial flora of the skin of the face has been extensively studied because of its possible central importance in the pathogenesis of acne (*see* Chapter 4). Essentially two species are found—the micrococci and *Corynebacterium (Proprionobacterium) acnes*. There are many antigenic types of the micrococci ('M' and 'S' strains) (Baird-Parker, 1963). The *Corynebacterium acnes* has also been recently subdivided by phage typing and it has been claimed that different phage types have differing capacities for lipolysis of triglycerides (Kellum et al., 1970).

REFERENCES

Baird-Parker A. C. (1963) A classification of micrococci and staphylococci based on physiological and biochemical tests. *J. Gen. Microbiol.* **30,** 409.

Borrie P. (1955) The state of the blood vessels of the face in rosacea. *Br. J. Dermatol.* **67,** 5.

Clayden J. R., Bell J. W. and Pollard P. (1974) Menopausal flushing: double blind trial of a non-hormonal medication. *Br. Med. J.* **1,** 409.

Ellis J. P., Marks R. and Perry B. J. (1970) Lymphatic function, the disappearance rate of ^{131}I albumin from the dermis. *Br. J. Dermatol.* **82,** 593.

Epstein E. H. and Epstein W. L. (1966) New cell formation in human sebaceous glands. *J. Invest. Dermatol.* **46,** 453.

Fox R. H., Goldsmith R. and Kidd D. J. (1962) Cutaneous vasomotor control in the human head, neck and upper chest. *J. Physiol. (Lond.)* **161,** 298.

Froese G. and Burton A. C. (1957) Heat losses from the human head. *J. Appl. Physiol.* **10**, 235.

Kellum R. E., Strangfeld K. and Ray L. T. (1970) Acne vulgaris. Studies in pathogenesis: triglyceride hydrolysis by corynebacterium acnes *in vitro*. *Arch. Dermatol.* **101**, 41.

Larson D. L., Coers C. R., Rodin A. E., Parcansky G. M., Corujo M. R. and Lewis S. R. (1967) Lymphatics of the upper and lower lip. A clinical and experimental study. *Am. J. Surg.* **114**, 525.

Marks R. and Dawber R. P. (1971) Skin surface biopsy: an improved technique for the examination of the horny layer. *Br. J. Dermatol.* **84**, 117.

Montagna W., Yun J. and Formisano V. (1964) Histology and cytochemistry of human skin: cholinesterase-containing nerves in face. *Arch. Dermatol.* **90**, 526.

Watkins P. J. (1973) Facial sweating after food: a new sign of diabetic autonomic neuropathy. *Br. Med. J.* **1**, 583.

Chapter 2

Rosacea

INTRODUCTION

Rosacea is a common disease. It accounts for approximately 2 per cent of new patients seen at St John's Hospital for Diseases of the Skin (Neves, 1966). It affects women more frequently than men though the quoted sex ratio varies according to the geographical situation of the particular author and the social milieu of his practice. Søbye (1950) remarked that the disease was particularly prone to occur in women between the ages of 30 and 50 and the ratio of women to men in his series was 3·3 : 1. Unfortunately, there are no reliable figures for either the true incidence or the real sex ratio for its occurrence in the community. Rosacea seems to be most common in the fourth and fifth decades, although it may be seen sometimes in patients in their early and mid-20's. It is doubtful whether true rosacea occurs in childhood though a child aged three with either rosacea or a disease simulating rosacea was shown at the St John's Hospital Dermatological Society (Pope, 1970) (*Fig.* 7). Other children with a rosacea-like eruption have been described by Savin et al. (1972).

The disease is characteristically a disorder of the fair-haired, blue-eyed 'Nordic type' and it is common in Scandinavia and North-west Europe generally. It is less common in individuals with darker complexions and is unusual in Asian peoples—although strangely enough it is quite common in some 'Red Indians' in the American mid-West (Everett, 1974). It is extremely rare in Negro individuals.

HISTORY

A fiery red complexion was linked by both Chaucer and Shakespeare to rumbustious living and overindulgence in alcoholic drinks. In *Henry IV*, *Part* 1, Falstaff taunts Bardolph with his red face and nose— 'I never see thy face but I think upon hell fire . . .' and '. . . but 'tis the nose of thee: thou art the knight of the burning lamp'. There are many similar references in Chaucer's 'General Prologue' to *The Canterbury*

number of synonyms for this disfiguring complaint; many such as 'rum nose' and *Eléphantiasis des buveurs* suggest that alcoholism is a predisposing cause. However, there is no evidence for this bit of folklore (Søbye, 1950; Marks et al., 1967). In contrast to rosacea itself, this affliction is perhaps ten or twenty times more common in men than women. It starts with mild persistent reddening of the tip of the nose, with prominent pilosebaceous orifices (*Fig.* 11). It progresses gradually with increasing craggy enlargement and a deepening of a variety of blue-red shades so that a grotesque state may eventually be reached (*Plate* 2B). The dilated hair follicles contain a foul-smelling mixture of keratinous debris and sebum which can be expressed by pressure on the nose. Sams (1932) described involvement of the chin in a similar but less florid process and Marks and Harcourt-Webster (1969) described another patient with the same condition. Rarely the forehead may become 'phymatous' too. I have seen thickening of the ear lobes in rosacea, although this does not seem to have quite the same basis, as oedema is the most prominent feature histologically in this complication.

Acker and Helwig (1967) described 5 patients in whom basal cell epitheliomata occurred with rhinophyma. On reviewing the literature they found 2 other cases of basal cell epithelioma and 3 examples of squamous cell carcinoma complicating rhinophyma.

Ocular Complications

Some affection of the eyes may be expected in approximately 50 per cent of patients with rosacea. Starr and McDonald (1969) found 58 per cent of their patients had ocular involvement. Conjunctivitis is by far the commonest ocular component of the rosacea complex and some conjunctival suffusion and mild discomfort of the eyes, not amounting to conjunctivitis, is seen in most patients with acute papular rosacea. Blepharitis, meibomian cysts, chalazion and styes are other ophthalmic complications similar to conjunctivitis, in that none is specific to rosacea. Their clinical course and treatment is the same as for the condition uncomplicated by rosacea. Episcleritis and iritis are other ophthalmic disorders accompanying rosacea, but they are rare (Borrie, 1953). More important is rosacea keratitis. This appears to be specific for this skin disease in contrast to the other eye conditions mentioned. Borrie (1953) found that it occurred relatively more frequently in men, although this was not the experience of Goldsmith, three-quarters of whose patients with keratitis were women (Goldsmith, 1953). Its development is not related to the severity of the facial eruption and it is not uncommon for it actually to precede the rash. It is painful, relapsing and may be relentlessly progressive, leading to scarring and even corneal perforation.

The cornea is affected from the periphery by encroaching blood vessels. Subepithelial cellular infiltrates develop and wedge-shaped opacities follow. It can be a very destructive process which is extremely troublesome to treat. Starr and McDonald (1969) found that 33 per cent of their rosacea patients showed corneal involvement, though Borrie (1953) found that only 3 per cent showed severe corneal changes. Interestingly, tetracycline has been found to be helpful for the keratitis as well as the rash (Marmion, 1969).

Lymphoedema

Apart from the facial swelling that may accompany acute inflammatory episodes, persistent boggy swelling is also occasionally seen. This mostly affects the periorbital tissues (*Fig.* 12), but other areas such as the forehead may be involved. It often causes difficulty in diagnosis as the accompanying rosacea may be mild. As with lymphoedema due to other causes, the swollen area is subject to episodes of acute inflammation with increased swelling, pain and tenderness. These often settle without treatment and there is little evidence that they are bacterial in origin as is often assumed. This complication, which for some reason seems to be more common in men, resists the most determined therapeutic efforts but may spontaneously improve.

Disseminated Rosacea

This term was given by Marks and Wilson Jones (1969) to patients with typical papular rosacea affecting the face, who developed the characteristic papular lesions of rosacea elsewhere on the body. Lesions seemed particularly prone to occur on the limbs in those patients (*Fig.* 13). However, two men with rosacea and rhinophyma who developed lesions in the presternal area were described by Rockl et al. (1969).

CLINICAL TYPES

Once the disease has developed, the tendency to have rosacea seems to persist for life. In some patients the development of persistent redness of the cheeks is followed by successive crops of papules and pustules with swelling, and they seem particularly prone to these episodes of inflammation.

In others the main features are an unchanging redness and telangiectasia, perhaps with an occasional papule. It is reasonable to divide the disease into the following clinical types:

1. Acute papular.
2. Erythemato-telangiectatic.
3. Lymphoedematous.

The acute papular type characteristically occurs in a patient who has noticed redness and telangiectasia for some time previously. It may start quite suddenly in the course of a few days. Left untreated it tends to improve gradually but the papules and swelling often recur. The erythemato-telangiectatic type develops slowly or sometimes is noted after a severe sunburn. It may persist indefinitely, perhaps becoming slightly more noticeable with the passage of time. Patients with this type may only present in the clinic when their rash develops into the acute papular variety. The lymphoedematous variety develops insidiously and persists with some fluctuation in the degree of swelling.

PATHOLOGY AND PATHOPHYSIOLOGY

Previously there has been too much emphasis on the presence of granulomatous inflammation in the dermis. Thus, the basic problems of the altered haemodynamics and tissue oedema have hardly been considered. Furthermore, too static an interpretation of biopsy material has also led to the view that the disorder is basically a folliculitis. In our own histopathological study only 15 of 74 biopsies of rosacea papules showed an abnormality of the pilosebaceous apparatus (Marks and Harcourt-Webster, 1969). Of these, 10 showed partial disruption of the follicular epithelium and polymorphonuclear leucocytic invasion of the substances of the pilosebaceous unit. This follicular disruption was the histological counterpart of the pustular lesions noted clinically. Follicular abnormalities did not seem to have major importance and perhaps were secondary events. Even when biopsies were cut serially, obliquely and horizontally, it was evident that much of the inflammation was entirely independent of the hair follicles. There is frequently a perifollicular cellular infiltrate, but on careful inspection it is seen to be related to the rich perivascular plexuses rather than the follicle itself (*Fig.* 14).

The dermal inflammatory cell infiltrate is often a striking feature in biopsies from rosacea papules. In very new papules there is a slight perivascular lymphohistiocytic cellular infiltrate set in an oedematous connective tissue stroma. In mature papules there is a dense mixed inflammatory cell infiltrate. The cell types seen include lymphocytes, histiocytes, plasma cells and occasional polymorphonuclear leucocytes. In addition, in 10–20 per cent a more granulomatous picture is seen with large histiocytes or epithelioid cells and foreign body giant cells (*Fig.* 15). Sometimes a tuberculoid granuloma is found. Although the pilosebaceous apparatus is infrequently involved, follicular disruption with abscess formation is seen in pustules (*Fig.* 15). During resolution and absorption of the destroyed follicle it is not uncommon to see a very dense inflammatory cell infiltrate which is granulomatous and often contains several giant cells. The inflammatory cell infiltrate is not tightly packed, as, for example, in lupus erythematosus, but is set in a loose oedematous connective tissue stroma in which there are prominent blood vessels.

The presence of tuberculoid granulomata in papular rosacea has been discussed by von Miescher (1943), Laymon (1951), Michelson (1958), Van Ketel (1958) and, more recently, by Mullenax and Kierland (1970). This melodramatic occurrence (in pathological terms) has captured the limelight and occupied too much attention.

A pathogenetically more significant change is seen in the upper dermis. Here there is oedematous, fragmented and disorganized connective tissue with prominent elastotic change. There is also considerable vessel dilatation in this zone of the dermis. Which of the affected vessels are blood vessels and which are dilated lymphatics is difficult to say with certainty. Many of them contain red cells (although lymphatics may occasionally also contain red cells), and it is unusual to see a condensation of elastic tissue around these enlarged channels or projecting endothelial cell nuclei. These observations favour the view that the channels represent a telangiectasia rather than a lymphangiectasia. In addition, it would seem reasonable that these vessels are the histological counterpart of the clinically evident telangiectasia. Elastotic change seems more extensive and more frequent in patients with rosacea (Marks and Harcourt-Webster, 1969) and this adds to the disorganization in the upper dermis (*Fig.* 16). This dystrophic process in the upper dermis, in failing to provide an adequate support for the vascular channels traversing it, allows them to dilate passively. Most of the observed vascular phenomena can be explained on the basis of passive dilatation of the vascular channels.

Apart from the histological picture of the peripheral lesions in disseminated rosacea (*see below*) and apart from their great size, the vessels are not inflamed or in other ways affected. However, as stated previously the vessels are frequently surrounded by oedematous stroma containing chronic inflammatory cells.

It is fair to say that although there is no single histological feature that is unique to rosacea, the changes described above when considered together are characteristic for it and should suggest the diagnosis in a biopsy of facial skin.

Rhinophyma

The microscopic picture depends on the stage of the disease reached. A gross sebaceous gland hyperplasia is often described as being characteristic, but is more often seen in the well-developed rhinophyma. In our own study the earliest changes observed seemed similar to those described for ordinary rosacea in that there was dermal oedema, a variable amount of chronic inflammatory cell infiltrate and disorganization in the upper dermis.

Disseminated Rosacea

Marks and Wilson Jones (1969) described the changes in the disseminated lesions in some detail. In brief, although the facial lesions of their patients had the same changes histopathologically as in typical rosacea the peripheral lesions were unusual. There appeared to be more active involvement of small blood vessels; they showed endothelial cell swelling and even fibrinoid necrosis. The presence of large and atypical monocytoid cells was noted in some lesions and in others there seemed to be a necrobiotic change in the connective tissue of the dermis.

DIFFERENTIAL DIAGNOSIS

Difficulty in diagnosis seldom arises, but there are some pitfalls that should be avoided. Rosacea must be distinguished from:
1. Seborrhoeic dermatitis.
2. Acne vulgaris.
3. Acne agminata.
4. Perioral dermatitis.
5. Systemic lupus erythematosus.
6. Polymorphic light eruption.
7. Dermatomyositis.
8. The malar flush of mitral stenosis.
9. The flush of the carcinoid syndrome.
10. Banal facial telangiectasia.
11. Haber's syndrome.
12. Sarcoidosis.
13. Facial erysipelas.
14. Suffusion of the face due to superior vena caval obstruction or polycythaemia.

Seborrhoeic dermatitis is characterized by scaling which is not often a feature of rosacea (unless overenthusiastically treated with preparations meant for acne). Furthermore, the areas involved are the nasolabial folds, the eyebrows, and in most patients the scalp (*see Fig.* 8).

Comedones, scars and cysts are not usually features of rosacea but are of *acne vulgaris*. In acne, lesions are scattered over the face, back and chest, and are not concentrated on the classical sites for rosacea. Occasionally a background of erythema develops on the face of a patient with severe persistent acne and then the differentiation can be difficult. It may be that because of the inflammation in the dermis the same basic change is occurring in the subpapillary venous plexus in these patients.

In *acne agminata* there are brownish-red papules around the eyes, on the eyelids, around the nose and on the upper lip; there is no background of erythema, no telangiectasia and no pustules.

The rash in *perioral dermatitis* is predominantly around the mouth, (*Fig. 8*) and consists of very small papules and pustules. The patient is characteristically a young woman and there is usually a background of slight pinkness only, and no telangiectasia.

The symmetrical erythema involving the cheeks and nose in a 'butterfly distribution' in acute *systemic lupus erythematosus* is uncommon. Patients with rosacea are often mistakenly referred to outpatient departments with this label. In SLE the patient is in general 'ill' and the erythema is unaccompanied by the other physical signs of rosacea.

Patients with a *polymorphic light eruption* complain that the rash occurs on other light-exposed areas besides the face. The rash is either eczematous or plaque-like and unlike rosacea.

The mauve hue or so-called 'heliotrope' discoloration of the eyelids and periocular skin in *dermatomyositis* should help distinguish this disorder. The presence of muscle weakness and erythema on the hands should also differentiate this disease.

The cyanotic tinged *malar flush* occurring over the upper part of cheeks in patients with mitral valve disease is not usually confused with rosacea.

The flushing and telangiectasia of the face in the *carcinoid syndrome* may cause more difficulty and according to Starr and McDonald (1969) can anyway be associated with rosacea.

Banal facial telangiectasia of mild degree is extremely common, but when extensive is much more unusual. It is then sometimes familial and anyway unassociated with the other physical signs of rosacea.

Haber's syndrome (Sanderson and Wilson, 1965) or 'familial rosacea-like eruption with intra-epidermal epithelioma' has been described in one family only.

Sarcoidosis may cause nasal swelling which could be confused with rhinophyma by the unwary. A micropapular variety occurring around the nose may also cause difficulty at times.

Facial erysipelas which causes a swollen red area may be symmetrical on the face, spreading across the nose, and on the cheeks, but the tenderness and heat of the affected area are characteristic for this infection.

The author has seen patients with *superior vena caval obstruction* referred with a diagnosis of rosacea even though the patients' faces were swollen and cyanotic in all areas, and there were distended neck veins. A similar mistake could be made in patients with *polycythaemia*.

AETIOLOGY AND PATHOGENESIS

No other skin disease has been so surrounded by folklore and mythology. An apt comment on the subject is that of Borrie: '. . . the wealth of unsubstantiated hypothesis on this subject varies from something alkaline in the stomach to something horrid in the cowshed' (Borrie, 1953).

The Gastro-intestinal Tract

Traditionally the development of rosacea has been associated with dietary excesses of one sort or another or with gastro-intestinal malfunction. In particular an excessive intake of alcoholic drinks, tea, coffee, spicy foods and other 'gastric irritants' have been supposed to predispose to the development of the disease. Detailed investigation into the dietary habits of rosacea patients has not confirmed any particular dietary anomaly (Søbye, 1950; Marks, 1968) and emphasizes the need for a critical approach. Hypochlorhydria was thought to be characteristic of rosacea (Brown, 1925; Eastwood, 1928; Epstein and Susnow, 1930). Later the limitations of 'fractional gastric analysis' and the dangers of uncontrolled observations were realized when Brown et al. (1935) reported that 'marked subacidity is not a feature peculiar to rosacea as was originally thought'. Interestingly this and similar observations did not stem the flow of dilute hydrochloric acid prescribed for this disorder.

Flatulent dyspepsia, constipation and diarrhoea have all been held to be more common in rosacea patients. Yet when a comparison was made between a group with rosacea and a matched control group no increase was found in symptoms referable to the gastro-intestinal tract (Marks et al., 1967). Gastroscopic examination of rosacea patients revealed 'evidence of gastritis' (Usher, 1941; Conrad et al., 1950). However, Fry (1968) could not confirm this finding using a gastroscope with fibre-optics. Gastric biopsies did not show any more abnormalities in rosacea patients than in matched controls (Marks et al., 1967).

The most recent round in this saga of enthusiastic 'thrust' and critical 'parry' has been the report of Watson et al. (1965) in which they found significant jejunal mucosal abnormalities in one-third of rosacea patients, and evidence of coeliac disease in 4 of 60. When a similar study was conducted in which the findings were compared with a control group of skin patients, no significant abnormalities could be detected in the rosacea group (Marks et al., 1967.)

A reason for the popular association between rosacea and the alimentary tract might be the more frequent flushing that rosacea patients experience to gastro-intestinal stimuli (Marks et al., 1967).

Psychosomatic Considerations

As with any chronic disfiguring disease of the face it would be strange if patients did not become depressed and disturbed. A mild and significant depressive tendency was the only psychiatric abnormality found in an investigation in which patients were asked 'standard' questions during interview and were submitted to a psychometric test (Marks, 1968). Similarly neither Søbye (1950) nor Whitlock (1961) found any particular personality disorder or psychiatric complaint in rosacea patients. Nonetheless the flushing has led many to speculate on the existence of a personality defect in rosacea patients (Obermayer, 1955; Plesch, 1962). The term 'morbid blushing' has been used by some in describing rosacea.

Demodex folliculorum

This mite lives predominantly in hair follicles of the head and neck. Its life cycle was elucidated by Spickett (1961). No definite role can be given to *Demodex* in the aetiology of any skin disease.

Many other mammalian species besides man are parasitized by their own variety of *Demodex*. In some animals, the organism is undoubtedly responsible for a skin disorder. In the demodectic mange of dogs, the *Demodex* can be seen to have disrupted the hair follicle and to lie within the dermis where it evokes an inflammatory response. In the marsupial mouse, a related mite is associated with benign skin tumours in which giant cell systems are seen (Nutting and Beerman, 1965).

The belief that *Demodex folliculorum* plays some role in the cause of rosacea stems from their frequent presence in great numbers in the disorder. They are easily demonstrable in KOH preparations of scrapings from many patients with papular rosacea (Brodie, 1952, found the infestation in 86 per cent of rosacea patients). Ayres and Ayres (1961) believed that there are two special varieties of rosacea caused by the *Demodex*, characterized by small scaly papules and a rapid clinical response to topical miticides. They term these 'pityriasis folliculorum' and 'acne rosacea *(Demodex)*'.

Russell (1962) and Spickett (1962) also believe that the *Demodex* plays a significant role in rosacea. This view is based on the presence of the organisms in the skin, albeit in increased numbers, without other supporting evidence. Although the mite is frequently seen in biopsy sections from rosacea, it is also seen in normal skin and in numerous disorders of the skin of the face. Follicles containing demodices are not the focal point of an inflammatory response (Marks and Harcourt-Webster, 1969) which one would reasonably expect if the mites are causing the disease. In addition, Robinson (1965) found no correlation between the responses of patients to a topical preparation containing 3 per cent sulphur and the presence of the organism as assessed histologically. Unfortunately there have been no studies as to whether *Demodex folliculorum* or its products can evoke an immunological response. Soluble antigens derived from the *Demodex* could diffuse across the follicle wall and produce a hypersensitivity response, but this hypothesis cannot be tested until a *Demodex* antigen is available. At the time of writing there is no good evidence for the involvement of this mite in the development of rosacea.

Climatic Exposure

Many rosacea patients complain bitterly that their rashes are made worse by exposure to the sun or to the cold wind. In addition the distribution of the eruption on the face is similar to that of a photo-dermatitis. Scandinavian dermatologists have been particularly impressed by the part played by exposure in the development of rosacea (Haxthausen, 1930: Søbye, 1950). Brodthagen (1955) treated patients with mepacrine and chloroquine and found that those patients who claimed that their rosacea was provoked by sunlight benefit by this treatment. However, he could not demonstrate any abnormal reaction to light in rosacea patients, nor could he induce rosacea at the sites of testing. Others have also failed to demonstrate any hypersensitivity to light on testing. As mentioned previously, individuals with blue eyes and fair hair are more prone to rosacea than those with dark com-plexions. In addition it appears that facial skin of rosacea patients is more prone to elastotic degeneration than similar skin from matched controls (Marks and Harcourt-Webster, 1969). Further information is needed on the effect of climatic factors other than sunlight on dermal connective tissue. In the writer's view, the dystrophy in the upper dermis may be due in some instances to climatic exposure, though what physical factor or factors are responsible is unknown.

Bacterial Infection

The situation is similar to that in acne. Pathogenic bacteria cannot be cultivated from surface swabs, or from biopsy specimens. In addition, Gram-stained biopsy sections did not reveal any abnormal collections of micro-organisms (Marks, 1968).

Reactivity to Vasoactive Substances

It has been suggested that the vascular phenomena in rosacea might be due to a changed reactivity to physiological vasoactive substances. However, Borrie (1955b) found no difference in reactivity to adrenaline, noradrenaline, histamine or acetyl choline in patients with rosacea compared to controls. No difference in the excretion of 5-hydroxyindole-acetic acid in the urine was found in rosacea patients compared to controls (Rowell and Summerscales, 1961). The possibility that bradykinin plays some role in the aetiology of this disorder was suggested by Starr and McDonald (1969), but there is no evidence for this.

Immunoglobulins

Recently immunoglobulins have been detected at the dermo-epidermal junction of approximately half the patients with rosacea (Baart de la Faille and Baart de la Faille Kuyper, 1969; Salo, 1970). The significance of these findings is difficult to interpret but may merely indicate the presence of a long-standing inflamed dermis. They certainly have not been detected in every series of patients examined by immunofluorescence methods (Abell et al., 1974).

Kinetics of the Inflammatory Reaction

The inflammation is markedly granulomatous at times in rosacea, and is always primarily a perivascular affair. The author investigated the cellular component of the inflammatory reaction by enzyme histochemical and autoradiographic techniques after injection of tritiated thymidine (Marks, 1973). 'Labelled' cells were found in the walls of and around the dilated blood vessels. The pattern of labelling did not suggest that the cellular infiltrate was primarily a hypersensitivity reaction but that there was a moderately high rate of cell death in the cellular infiltrate.

Riboflavine

It is of historical interest to note that because of the superficial similarity of rosacea keratitis to riboflavine deficiency in animals it was suggested that riboflavine metabolism might be concerned in the aetiology of rosacea (Johnson and Eckardt, 1940).

Conclusion

The cause of rosacea is unknown. It is better to admit our ignorance than to subscribe to hypotheses for which there is no evidence. Nevertheless, it seems possible that the dermal disorganization described above is important in the production of a persistently dilated subpapillary venous plexus, and that this is one step in the *pathogenesis of rosacea.*

TREATMENT

Papular rosacea responds to the systemic administration of the tetracycline group of antibiotics (Sneddon, 1966). The response is often more dramatic and less equivocal than in acne. As in acne improvement starts between the third and fourth week of administration. A convenient treatment regime is to start with tetracycline 250 mg three times per day for the first week and then twice daily till there are no further papules. At this point the dose is reduced to 250 mg daily for the next 2 weeks and then 250 mg alternate days for the subsequent 2 weeks. This treatment has only a marginal effect on the background of erythema although this may improve slowly after the acute papular episode has subsided. Other antibiotics such as ampicillin and erythromycin do not appear to be as effective.

In one trial one group of patients was given tetracycline, a second group was given ampicillin and a third was given a placebo. The response was measured by counting the numbers of papules and pustules in predetermined areas of the cheek and the forehead. The group treated with tetracycline did extremely well compared to the other two groups but to the writer's surprise the group treated with ampicillin also made a small but significant improvement (Marks and Ellis, 1971).

Why the tetracyclines should work so well and the way in which they work are further mysteries in the complex story of rosacea.

The time interval before improvement and the small dose with which the development of papules can be suppressed suggest that perhaps these compounds have an effect other than an antibiotic one. This suggestion is reinforced by the comparative lack of effectiveness of other antibiotics and the failure to find significant pathogenic bacteria associated with the clinical lesions. (For further discussion of this problem see Chapter 4.)

Topical Applications

There is no place for the use of the potent topical corticosteroids in rosacea. They certainly seem to 'damp down' the inflammatory aspects of the disease but only during continued application. Because of the immediate worsening when they are no longer used, patients often become dependent on them. After prolonged use on the face they have the paradoxical effect of causing increased redness and telangiectasia (Sneddon, 1969). Sneddon (1973) examined the effect of hydrocortisone-17-butyrate in rosacea and found it not to be associated with this unwanted effect. The explanation for this harmful result is probably that the steroids by their 'wasting' effect on connective tissue increase the dermal dystrophy and hence the tendency to dilatation of the subpapillary venous plexus.

Sulphur- and ichthyol-containing preparations are supposed to be helpful but any therapeutic value they have is marginal. There is no harm in prescribing 2 per cent ichthyol in simple aqueous or oily creams—certainly it helps prevent patients applying corticosteroids.

Treatment of Rhinophyma

Tetracyclines are slightly helpful in that they stop papule and pustule formation. The swelling and discoloration are not influenced by tetracycline administration. The appearance can be considerably improved by surgery. The surgical procedure that is most helpful is 'shaving'—re-epithelialization taking place from the enormously hypertrophied hair follicles (Odou and Odou, 1961). Other surgical manœuvres, including formal plastic reconstruction, are described but do not appear to be as satisfactory as 'shaving'.

Treatment of Rosaceous Lymphoedema

This is the most difficult complication of rosacea to treat. Protracted courses of tetracyclines have the effect of preventing acute episodes of inflammation but have no or little effect on the persistent swelling. Søbye (1950) recommended massage, but this does not seem to be of any real value. Occasionally for periocular lymphoedema, surgery can be helpful by removing the lymphoedematous 'bags' that form. The only bright aspect to this type of rosacea is that slow natural resolution seems to take place in some patients.

REFERENCES

Abell E., Black M. M. and Marks R. (1974) Immunoglobulin and complement deposits in the skin in inflammatory facial dermatoses—an immunofluorescent study. *Br. J. Dermatol.* **91**, 281.

Acker D. W. and Helwig E. B. (1967) Rhinophyma with carcinoma. *Arch. Dermatol.* **95**, 250.

Ayres S. jun. and Ayres S. III (1961) Demodectic eruptions (demodecidosis) in the human. *Arch. Dermatol.* **83**, 816.

Baart de la Faille H. and Baart de la Faille Kuyper E. H. (1969) Immunofluorescent studies of the skin in rosacea. *Dermatologica* **139**, 49.

Borrie J. P. (1953) Rosacea with special reference to its ocular manifestations. *Br. J. Dermatol.* **65**, 458.

Borrie J. P. (1955a) The state of the blood vessels in the face in rosacea. *Br. J. Dermatol.* **67**, 73.

Borrie J. P. (1955b) The state of the blood vessels of the face in rosacea. *Br. J. Dermatol.* **67**, 5.

Brodie R. C. E. (1952) Rosacea: the role of *Demodex folliculorum*. *Aust. J. Dermatol.* **3**, 149.

Brodthagen H. (1955) Mepacrine and chloroquine in the treatment of rosacea. *Br. J. Dermatol.* **67**, 421.

Brown W. H. (1925) Some observations on the fractional method of gastric analysis in diseases of the skin. *Br. J. Dermatol.* **37**, 213.

Brown W. H., Smith M. S. and McLachlan A. D. (1935) Fractional gastric analysis in diseases of the skin. Further observations in 316 cases, with special reference to rosacea. *Br. J. Dermatol.* **47**, 181.

Conrad A. H., Kenamore B. D. and Lonergan W. N. (1950) Results of gastroscopic examinations in patients with acne rosacea. *South. Med. J.* **43**, 631.

Eastwood S. R. (1928) Gastric secretion and other digestive factors in rosacea. *Br. J. Dermatol.* **40**, 91, 148.

Epstein N. and Susnow D. (1930) Acne rosacea with particular reference to gastric secretion. *Calif. East. Med.* **35**, 118.

Everett, M. A. (1974) Personal communication.

Fry L. (1968) Gastro-camera studies in rosacea. *Br. J. Dermatol.* **80**, 737.

Goldsmith A. J. B. (1953) The ocular manifestations of rosacea. *Br. J. Dermatol.* **65**, 448.

Haxthausen H. (1930) Changes in the skin vessels from protracted action of climatic factors and their significance in various skin diseases. *Br. J. Dermatol.* **42**, 105.

Johnson L. V. and Eckardt R. E. (1940) Rosacea keratitis and conditions with vascularization of cornea treated with riboflavin. *Arch. Ophthalmol.* **23**, 899.

Laymon C. W. (1951) Lupoid rosacea. *Arch. Dermatol.* **63**, 409.

Lewis Sir T. (1927) *The Blood-vessels of the Human Skin and their Responses.* London, Shaw.

Marks R. (1968) Concepts in the pathogenesis of rosacea. *Br. J. Dermatol.* **80**, 170.

Marks R. (1973) Histogenesis of the inflammatory component of rosacea. *Proc. R. Soc. Med.* **66**, 742.

Marks R., Beard R. J., Clark M. L., Kwok M. and Robertson W. B. (1967) Gastro-intestinal observation in rosacea. *Lancet* **1**, 739.

Marks R. and Ellis J. (1971) Comparative effectiveness of tetracycline and ampicillin in rosacea. A controlled trial. *Lancet* **2**, 1049.

Marks R. and Harcourt-Webster N. (1969) Histopathology of rosacea. *Arch. Dermatol.* **100**, 683.

Marks R. and Wilson Jones E. (1969) Disseminated rosacea. *Br. J. Dermatol.* **81**, 16.

Marmion V. J. (1969) Tetracyclines in the treatment of ocular rosacea. *Proc. R. Soc. Med.* **62**, 11.

Michelson H. E. (1958) Does the rosacea-like tuberculid exist? *Arch. Dermatol.* **78**, 681.

Von Miescher G. (1943) Rosacea und rosacea-aehnliche Tuberkulide. *Dermatologica* **88**, 150.

Mullenax M. G. and Kierland R. R. (1970) Granulomatous rosacea. *Arch. Dermatol.* **101**, 206.

Neves H. (1966) Incidence of skin diseases 1952–1965. *Trans. St John's Hosp. Dermatol. Soc.* **52**, 255.

Nutting W. B. and Beerman H. (1965) Atypical giant cells in antechinus stuartii due to demodicid mites. *J. Invest. Dermatol.* **45**, 504.

Obermayer M. E. (1955) *Psychocutaneous Medicine.* Springfield, Ill., Thomas, p. 280.

Odou B. L. and Odou E. R. (1961) Rhinophyma. *Am. J. Surg.* **102**, 3.

Plesch E. (1962) A Rorschach study of rosacea and morbid blushing. *Acta Psychother. Psychosom. Orthop.* **10**, 45.

Pope F. M. (1970) Juvenile rosacea, steroid facies. *Trans. St John's Hosp. Dermatol. Soc.* **56**, 206.

Robinson T. W. E. (1965) *Demodex folliculorum* and rosacea. *Arch. Dermatol.* **92**, 542.

Rockl H., Germon J., Schropl F. and Scherer M. (1969) Rosacea mit extrafacialer Lokalisation. *Hautarzt* **8**, 348.

Rowell N. R. and Summerscales J. W. (1961) Urinary excretion of 5-hydroxyindole-acetic acid in rosacea. *J. Invest. Dermatol.* **36**, 405.

Russell B. F. (1962) Some aspects of the biology of the epidermis. *Br. Med. J.* **1**, 815.

Salo O. P. (1970) SLE like deposition of immunoglobulins in the skin in rosacea. *Ann. Clin. Res.* **2**, 28.

Sams W. M. (1932) Rhinophyma, with unusual involvement of the chin. *Arch. Dermatol.* **26**, 834.

Sanderson K. V. and Wilson H. T. H. (1965) Haber's syndrome. Familial rosacea-like eruption with intraepidermal epitheliomata. *Br. J. Dermatol.* **77**, 1.

Savin J., Marks R. and Alexander S. (1972) A rosacea-like eruption in children. *Br. J. Dermatol.* **87**, 425.

Sneddon I. (1966) A clinical trial of tetracycline in rosacea. *Br. J. Dermatol.* **78**, 649.

Sneddon I. (1969) Adverse effect of topical fluorinated corticosteroids in rosacea. *Br. Med. J.* **1**, 671.

Sneddon I. (1973) A trial of hydrocortisone butyrate in the treatment of rosacea and perioral dermatitis. *Br. J. Dermatol.* **89**, 505.

Søbye P. (1950) Aetiology and pathogenesis of rosacea. *Acta Derm. Venereol.* **30**, 137.

Spickett S. G. (1961) Studies on *Demodex folliculorum* Simon (1842). *Parasitology* **51**, 181.

Spickett S. G. (1962) Aetiology of rosacea. *Br. Med. J.* **1**, 1625.

Starr P. A. J. and McDonald A. (1969) Oculocutaneous aspects of rosacea. *Proc. R. Soc. Med.* **62**, 9.

Usher B. (1941) Gastroscopic observations in rosacea. *Arch. Dermatol. Syph.* **44**, 251.

Van Ketel W. G. (1958) Rosacea-like tuberculid of Lewandowski. *Dermatologica* **116**, 201.

Watson W. C., Paton E. and Murray D. (1965) Small-bowel disease in rosacea. *Lancet* **2**, 47.

Whitlock F. A. (1961) Psychosomatic aspects of rosacea. *Br. J. Dermatol.* **73**, 137.

Chapter 3

Perioral Dermatitis

INTRODUCTION

In 1957 Frumess and Lewis reported, under the term 'light-sensitive seborrhoeide', a new entity characteristically occurring in young women and restricted to the face. Since then there have been several reports of what seems to be the same disorder and which has been called 'facial dermatitis of unknown cause' by Kaufman (1965), 'perioral dermatitis' by Mihan and Ayres (1964) and 'rosacea-like dermatitis' by Stiegleder and Strempel (1968). The first report from Europe was by Hjorth et al. in 1968 and similar patients have also been seen in Australia by Finley (1969). A particularly interesting feature of this disorder is its apparently recent appearance (or at least recognition). At one time it seemed relatively common (accounting for 0·5 per cent of new patients seen at St John's Hospital, London, in 1969), but it is my impression that it is now decreasing in incidence. Whether it is an entirely new entity or a variant of either seborrhoeic dermatitis or rosacea is uncertain. It is certain, however, that it is a common clinical problem that merits the attention of general practitioners and dermatologists alike.

All are agreed that perioral dermatitis is most often seen in young women. The average age in the series of Hjorth et al. was 29·6 years and it was 34 in the patients of van Dijk and co-workers (1970). All 62 patients in Kaufman's series were women whose ages ranged from 11 to 74 (Kaufman, 1965). Steigleder (1970) has found a similar age distribution though his youngest patient was 3! This disorder is uncommon in men, perhaps accounting for between 5 and 10 per cent of patients.

CLINICAL FEATURES

Definition

A persistent erythematous eruption composed of tiny papules and papulopustules distributed primarily around the mouth and not responsive to topical treatments.

Symptoms

Young women with this disorder are upset by its appearance though, probably because of its shorter duration and lesser extent, they appear less depressed than do patients with rosacea. It is occasionally itchy but a burning or smarting type of discomfort is more often described.

Signs

The basic lesion is a small pink papule 1–3 mm in diameter (*Plate* 3A) that sometimes looks translucent and almost vesicular. There is usually a background of diffuse pinkness in the area as well. The sites affected are shown in *Fig.* 8. Although the disorder is markedly 'perioral' and the chin, upper lip and nasolabial grooves are most severely affected (*Fig.* 17), a few papules may stray outside these areas to involve the sides of the nose and the glabella. A frequent finding is a clear uninvolved zone a few millimetres wide, immediately adjacent to the lips (*Fig.* 18). The rash varies slightly from day to day but complete spontaneous remission seems to be uncommon. The few men that do develop this condition seem to be more extensively affected (*Plate* 3B).

Premenstrual exacerbation as seen in acne is not common in perioral dermatitis. Exposure to the sun seems to aggravate the rash in some patients (*see below* p. 28) but there does not seem to be a marked seasonal variation in its incidence (*Fig.* 19). Patients with perioral dermatitis do not seem especially prone to either acne or, as has been suggested, dandruff and seborrhoeic dermatitis. In fact, these young women seem completely fit apart from their facial rash.

HISTOPATHOLOGY

There are few published reports on the pathology of this complaint. Kaminsky et al. (1966) and Hjorth et al. (1968) state that mild inflammatory changes are present, especially around the follicles. Steigleder (1970) thought that there was a histological similarity to rosacea. Marks and Black (1971) examined biopsies from 26 patients and did not find the characteristic oedema, upper dermal disorganization or focal granulomatous infiltrate that is so often seen in rosacea. In addition, in more than half of the biopsies examined there were mild eczematous changes (*Fig.* 20) in contrast to rosacea in which epidermal changes are uncommon. There were areas of spongiosis in the follicular epithelium in more than two-thirds of the specimens (*Fig.* 21) and often the eczematous changes in the interfollicular epithelium seemed to begin in or near a hair follicle. This spongiotic change was accompanied by invasion of the involved area of the follicles by lymphocytes and histiocytes. Apart from a small amount of infiltrate of chronic inflammatory cells scattered perivascularly, no other abnormalities were noted. A significant number of micro-organisms was not found in Gram-stained preparations.

AETIOLOGY

Many believe that this disorder is not a true entity but is merely a type of rosacea. However, there are a number of reasons for believing that it is not part of the rosacea complex:

- *a.* The lack of the characteristic persistent erythema, oedema and telangiectasia of rosacea indicates a basic difference in the patho-physiology of the two complaints.
- *b.* Perioral dermatitis occurs in a younger age group and is relatively less common in men than is rosacea.
- *c.* The ocular component of rosacea is not seen in perioral dermatitis.
- *d.* The histopathology of rosacea is quite distinct from that seen in perioral dermatitis.

There is one unexplained similarity between the two conditions, however, in that both respond in the same dramatic way to treatment with the tetracyclines.

The distribution in the nasolabial grooves and around the mouth has suggested a relationship to seborrhoeic dermatitis (whatever that is!). The only evidence in support of this has been the frequent presence of eczema in biopsies from patients with perioral dermatitis.

Most authors have concluded that perioral dermatitis is a separate entity and have considered the following possible causes.

1. *Allergic Contact Dermatitis.* Extensive patch testing has been performed in patients but no significant hypersensitivities were detected. Various cosmetics and toothpastes have been suspected but all were blameless when it came to formal patch testing (Cronin E. and Marks R., unpublished observations). However, Steigleder (1970) has found that some patients have had positive patch tests to the peel of citrus fruits or to toothpastes. Whether these were primary irritant reactions or hypersensitivity reactions is not known.

2. *Primary Irritant Dermatitis.* Patients have been questioned as to their use of such articles as paper handkerchiefs and their usual brands of soap, without any central theme emerging. It has also been suggested that the disorder is due to frequent contact with 'the boy friend's stubbly chin'. This attempt at attributing its sudden increase in incidence to the 'permissive society' has not met with approval from the few men and the many respectable ladies with perioral dermatitis!

3. *Moniliasis or Bacterial Infection.* Repeated examination of scrapings from affected sites has not revealed the presence of *Candida* species and bacterial swabs have only shown the normal flora for this area (Author,

1971, unpublished observations). Gram-stained histological preparations have not revealed significant numbers of bacteria in or near the
hair follicle. The reason for the good response to the tetracyclines is
unexplained. However, Beetz et al. (1973) found that they were able to
grow a Gram-negative fusiform bacillus from 47 of 69 patients but
from none of 33 controls with other papulopustular conditions on the
face. In addition, there are two other reports that should be mentioned.
Firstly, Oehlschlaegel et al. (1971) found that all their patients with
perioral dermatitis had a positive candida skin test and that 18 out of
24 patients gave a positive result to various bacterial antigens. Their
patients responded to topical nystatin or amphotericin. Secondly there
is the report of Bradford and Montes (1972) who cultivated *Candida
albicans* from their 32 patients and who found that their patients'
rashes cleared after treatment with nystatin topically. I find it difficult
to account for the findings in the above three reports as they do
not accord with the results of our studies or those of many other
groups.

4. *Hormonal Factors.* Premenstrual exacerbation occurred in 7 of
Finley's 39 patients and in 8 of the 38 female patients of Hjorth et al.
These are uncontrolled observations and it is possible that any aggra-
vation seen is non-specific. The high proportion of perioral dermatitis
patients taking the contraceptive pill has been often discussed. However, comparison must be made with the proportion of women of this
age group in the population at large also on 'the pill' before conclusions
can be drawn.

5. *Malabsorption.* Kaminsky et al. (1966) have suggested the
possibility of intestinal malabsorption in patients with perioral
dermatitis. There seems to be little evidence in favour of this suggestion.

6. *Topical Fluorinated Corticosteroids.* There can be few patients today
referred to the dermatologist who have not been given potent topical
corticosteroids to use at some stage. This certainly applies to patients
with perioral dermatitis and Verbov and Abell (1969) have suggested
that these preparations play an important role in the aetiology of the
disease. However, this view is not acceptable, as Rook et al. (1972) and
the writer have seen patients with perioral dermatitis before treatment
by topical steroid preparations.

7. *Light Sensitivity.* Frumess and Lewis (1957) originally described
this condition as 'light-sensitive seborrhoeide'. Many of their patients
complained that sunlight brought on or aggravated their rash. These
authors claimed that their patients were helped by antimalarials and
other measures protecting them from sunlight. No other author has
been convinced of the association with sun exposure and indeed some
patients claim that the condition is improved after sunbathing. Solar
elastosis is not a marked feature in biopsies of perioral dermatitis as it is

in rosacea, and connective tissue disorganization is similarly not a histological feature of perioral dermatitis. The author knows of no investigation that has undertaken formal light testing in this group of patients.

8. It is of considerable interest that the disease has become recognized primarily in the 'affluent society'. This is true both for the communities in which it has appeared and for the individuals who develop the disorder. The disease was first recognized in the U.S.A. in the mid-1950's and later spread to involve many other industrialized societies.

DIFFERENTIAL DIAGNOSIS

Perioral dermatitis must be distinguished from

1. Rosacea.
2. Acne.
3. Seborrhoeic dermatitis.
4. Allergic contact dermatitis.
5. *Erythrose péribuccale* of Brocq.

1. *Rosacea.* The lack of persistent erythema, of swelling and of telangiectasia in perioral dermatitis are the most important points in its separation from rosacea. The distribution of the eruption is also markedly different.

2. *Acne.* There are no comedones, cysts or inflamed papules in perioral dermatitis.

3. *Seborrhoeic Dermatitis.* There may be some difficulty in distinguishing this condition from perioral dermatitis if its distribution is predominantly facial. Other areas, such as the scalp, retro-auricular folds and eyebrows, are usually involved and scaling is a more prominent feature in seborrhoeic dermatitis. In addition, perioral dermatitis does not respond to topical preparations, whereas there is an improvement in seborrhoeic dermatitis when treated in this way.

4. *Allergic Contact Dermatitis.* Hypersensitivity to a constituent of lipstick such as eosin or lanolin produces a cheilitis and not the picture of perioral dermatitis. Allergic contact dermatitis to nail varnish or plants may affect the perioral area asymmetrically as well as other areas on the face.

5. *'Erythrose péribuccale' of Brocq.* This eruption is characterized by well-defined brown or pink macular areas, varying in shade from day to day around the mouth in young women. It was described by Brocq in 1923 but does not now seem to be diagnosed often in this country.

TREATMENT

Perioral dermatitis responds to the tetracyclines in the same way as rosacea. A suitable course of treatment is oxytetracycline 250 mg t.d.s. for 1 week then 250 mg b.d. until there is clearing of all papules (usually in 2–4 weeks). The same dose should then be continued for 2 weeks and then reduced to 250 mg daily for a further 2 weeks before stopping. Luckily there does not seem to be the same tendency for repeated attacks as there is in rosacea. There are no published controlled data concerning the response to this treatment but D. S. Wilkinson and N. Hjorth (personal communications) now share this view as to the response of the condition to the tetracyclines. There is no information as to the possible mode of action of the tetracyclines.

In general, topical applications are to be avoided. Many seem to aggravate the condition. Some potent topical corticosteroids seem to suppress it partially so long as they are used but allow a severe 'rebound' flare when stopped. (Warning should be given about this possibility after stopping topical corticosteroids.) It is worth while to prescribe aqueous cream BP as a palliative (if only to stop the patient using other local applications). The same caution as to eventual atrophy and telangiectasia after prolonged use of potent topical corticosteroids applies here as it does in rosacea.

REFERENCES

Beetz H. M., Schubert E. and Rockl H. (1973) Über die Bedeutung von Bakterien bei den sogenannter Periorale Dermatitis. *Hautarzt* **24**, 220.

Bradford L. G. and Montes L. F. (1972) Perioral dermatitis and *Candida albicans*. *Arch. Dermatol.* **105**, 892.

Brocq (1923) L'érythrose pigmentée péribuccale. *Presse Méd.* 22 August 1923, p. 727.

Finley A. G. (1969) Perioral dermatitis. *Aust. J. Dermatol.* **10**, 140.

Frumess G. M. and Lewis H. M. (1957) Light-sensitive seborrhoide. *Arch. Dermatol.* **75**, 245.

Hjorth N., Osmundsen P., Rook A. J., Wilkinson D. S. and Marks R. (1968) Perioral dermatitis. *Br. J. Dermatol.* **80**, 307.

Kaminsky A., Gaidamak D. and Resnik R. (1966) Dermatitis perioral. *Información dermatológica*, No. 19, 1965. *Cuadernos de dermatología* **3**, 161.

Kaufman W. H. (1965) Facial dermatitis of unknown cause. *JAMA* **192**, 252.

Marks R. and Black M. M. (1971) Perioral dermatitis. A histopathological study of 26 cases. *Br. J. Dermatol.* **84**, 242.

Mihan R. and Ayres S. jun. (1964) Perioral dermatitis. *Arch. Dermatol.* **89**, 803.

Oehlschlaegel G., Dungemann H., Schnabel P. and Lagally G. (1971) Zur Bedeutung von Hefeinfektionen in der Aktivpathogenese der Perioralen Dermatitis. *Hautarzt* **22**, 489.

Rook A., Wilkinson D. S. and Ebling F. J. C. (1972) *Textbook of Dermatology*, 2nd ed. Oxford, Blackwell Scientific.

Sneddon I. (1973) A trial of hydrocortisone butyrate in the treatment of rosacea and perioral dermatitis. *Br. J. Dermatol.* **89**, 505.

Steigleder G. K. (1970) Rosacea-like dermatitis (perioral dermatitis). *German Medical Monthly* **15**, 1.
Steigleder G. K. and Strempel A. (1968) Rosacea-artige Dermatitis des Gesichts: 'Periorale dermatitis'. *Hautarzt* **19**, 492.
van Dijk E., Kalsbeck G. H. and Verburgh-Van der Zwan N. (1970) Perioral dermatitis. *Dermatologica* **140**, 291.
Verbov J. and Abell E. (1969) Iatrogenic dermatitis. *Br. Med. J.* **4**, 621.

Chapter 4

Acne

INTRODUCTION

It is no accident that this is the longest chapter in this book. Acne is one of the commonest skin diseases, if not the commonest. It accounted for 8 per cent, on average, of new patients seen at St John's Hospital for Diseases of the Skin in the years 1960–9. In addition, investigators have made a great effort to understand this condition better in the past two decades, and this work will be discussed.

Few adolescents reach mature years without developing at least a few acne spots; between 30 and 50 per cent of youngsters between the ages of 10 and 19 are affected (Rook et al., 1972). Munro-Ashman (1963) found that 57 per cent of the boys in a public school were affected by acne (84 per cent of these cases were classified as mild). The age at which most were affected was 16. Damon (1957) found that 40 per cent of 400 soldiers in the United States Army had some acne. Of these 44 per cent were between 17 and 19 years old, 39 per cent were between 20 and 24 and 24 per cent were between 25 and 29. Similar findings were recorded by Forbes (1946) in the British Army.

The term 'physiological' is often applied to mild acne because of its frequency in the population. However, this term should not lull the clinician into a submissive state, as what appears 'physiological' to him is often a source of extreme anguish to the bearer of the spots. Although adolescence is the peak period for the appearance of acne, it is not very uncommon for patients to develop (for the first time) lesions in their 20's or even in the fourth decade. Certainly, it is incorrect to think of acne as being essentially a 'punishment for teenagers'.

There is little information concerning the distribution of acne in the various racial groups. Although none seems exempt, it appears that some populations are more affected than others. Caucasians are probably more severely and frequently affected than the Negro peoples.

The Anglo-Saxon is perhaps more prone to bad acne than Nordic or Mediterranean types, but Damon (1957) stated that in his series acne was probably not significantly associated with ancestry among white soldiers. However, there really is insufficient information on these points.

It is frequently said that boys are more severely affected than girls and certainly the worst cases of cystic acne seem to occur in young men. Men need not feel too aggrieved at this as women seem more prone to develop acne in the third and fourth decades and, furthermore, this late onset type of acne is also very persistent and often difficult to treat.

DEFINITION

Acne may be defined as follows: A disorder characterized by seborrhoea and obstruction of hair follicles with horny accumulations, and often complicated by the development of inflammatory lesions including papules, pustules and cysts of the face, neck, shoulders and chest.

CLINICAL PICTURE

Lesions

The following lesions may be seen in acne:
1. Comedones.
2. 'Whiteheads'.
3. Papules.
4. Pustules.
5. Cysts.
6. Scars: (*a*) 'Ice pick' and shallow 'pock'; (*b*) pits; (*c*) keloid and hypertrophic.

Comedones

These black-tipped tiny prominences are commonly seen in the less severe types of acne, and are often accompanied by marked oiliness of the skin. They seem less numerous when the acne is serious and when there is extensive inflammation. They mostly occur around the nose and forehead (*Fig.* 22), where there are many sebaceous follicles, but they are also common on the back and may be seen on any hairy area. They are composed of inspissated sebum and keratinous debris, and often contain small vellus hairs also.

The cause of the blackened tip of the otherwise grey-white comedo plug is interesting. 'Ingrained' dirt does not appear to be the answer. 'Oxidation' of some of the fatty constituents was accepted as the cause for some time but this also appears incorrect. Melanin is known to accumulate in follicle mouths and this accounts for the major part of the blackening. Blair and Lewis (1970) reviewed the subject and examined comedones macroscopically and histochemically themselves. They found granules at the tip of comedones that gave the staining reactions of melanin. They also found that there was a good correlation between the depth of colour of the comedo and the pigmentation of the surrounding skin. Why only the tip is coloured black is less certain. Strauss and Kligman (1960) divide comedones into the 'open' and the 'closed' varieties. The former give rise to the traditional blackhead and are harmless. The latter are dangerous as their follicular openings are very small and the follicle is more liable to rupture and cause an inflammatory lesion. Thus, in this concept the blackhead is only a sign of acne, but it may be accompanied by invisible comedones, which give rise to more serious lesions. Comedones may fluoresce red in ultraviolet light from coproporphyrin III produced by intrinsic *Corynebacteria acnes* (Cornelius and Ludwig, 1967).

Whiteheads

There is no adequate term for the small white non-inflammatory papules that occur most frequently on the cheeks and forehead. They represent blocked pilosebaceous follicles and are really another type of comedo. They are frequently seen accompanying blackheads and are especially common on the cheeks and forehead.

Papules

As most readers will recall from personal experience, acne papules are tender, which adds to the patient's discomfort. These lesions vary in size and are usually a dusky-red in colour. They are not often regularly hemispherical and may even be oblong in shape. Thus, they differ markedly from typical rosacea papules. Acne papules may last a long time, and before they finally disappear they may leave a dusky-red macule or a small firm fibrotic nodule.

The eruption of new papules is a good index of the activity of the disease and of the effectiveness of treatment.

Pustules

White or yellowish pustules (1–2 mm in diameter) may develop around comedones on pre-existing papules or on otherwise normal skin. They seem particularly common on the chin, forehead and back.

Cysts

These are the least common but the most serious manifestation of acne. They are the most stubborn type of lesion to treat, the most unsightly, and the most likely to lead to unpleasant scarring. The term 'cyst' is inaccurate; they do not have a proper lining epithelium and are in reality cold abscesses. These lesions are particularly common along the lower jaw, around the temple, on the cheeks (*Plate* 4A; *Fig.* 23) and on the upper part of the back. They vary greatly in size and may reach several centimetres in diameter. Their shape is often irregular and their tenderness seems to depend on the tension of their contents. Occasionally they spontaneously discharge a greyish or creamy pus, but if left to their own devices they gradually flatten to leave a variable degree of scar. They seem spontaneously to improve, and then may worsen. They are associated with a variable degree of inflammation in the surrounding skin.

Scars

The commonest types of scarring seen are: (*a*) the shallow pock type of scar; (*b*) pitted scars (*Fig.* 24). Unfortunately, these scars are often seen on the cheeks and are the cause of considerable unhappiness. They may result from the inflammatory papules of acne. The pitted areas represent pilosebaceous canals permanently dilated by fibrosis. These types of scars tend to become less prominent with passing years but never really disappear.

The most disfiguring type of scarring is (*c*) the keloidal variety seen particularly on the front of the chest, the shoulders and the back of the neck (*Fig.* 25). Keloidal 'bridging' is sometimes seen, especially when cysts have been incised and are allowed to heal by granulation. When deep papules and some cysts resolve they may leave a small firm nodule. These nodular lesions are not usually permanent and gradually flatten over several months.

Clinical Patterns

There is considerable overlap between the various types of acne but the patterns mentioned below are sufficiently distinctive to merit description.

1. *Superficial Acne*

In this group of patients inflammatory lesions are not prominent and are trivial when present. There are many comedones and a few small papules and pustules (*Plate* 4B). The outlook for these patients is extremely good, and their acne is usually a transient affair lasting a few months only.

2. *Papulopustular Acne*

This is the commonest pattern of acne seen in hospital outpatient practice, and it is characterized by the appearance of inflammatory papules and pustules. The severity and extent are extremely variable, ranging from the appearance of several tender papules on the forehead or back of neck to the profuse outbreak of papules and pustules affecting the face, shoulders and front of chest (*Fig. 24b*). Characteristically, the course of this type of acne is remittent and unpredictable. This type can lead to pitted scarring.

3. *Cystic Acne* (Conglobate Acne)
Cysts may be seen in association with profuse papular lesions, particularly round the cheeks (*Fig. 23*) and the back (*Fig. 25*), on the back of the neck (*Fig. 26*), the lower jaw, over the shoulders and on the front of the chest. Less commonly, they may be seen as the predominant lesion. Cysts may be reddened, tender and inflamed, or there may be no obvious inflammation. Cystic acne is also notoriously fickle in its clinical course. This type of acne is one of the most distressing dermatological conditions as far as disfigurement is concerned. A particularly severe type of cystic acne with draining sinuses and scarring is sometimes seen on the face and is then called 'pyoderma faciale.'

4. *Acne Keloid of the Back of the Neck*
Sometimes the back of the neck is affected by severe acne scars without much acne elsewhere. The appearance is characteristic and the condition may be compounded by manual interference by the patient (*Fig. 26*).

5. *Juvenile Acne*
The occurrence of a few acneiform spots on the cheeks of infants from 1 to 5 years of age is a not infrequent event (*Fig. 27*). It is uncommon for the lesions to be very inflamed or to be present in large numbers. Cystic lesions are virtually unknown in juvenile acne. Shallow pock-type scars are quite often seen, but are more often the result of enthusiastic excoriation rather than the acne lesions themselves. Comedones and small papules are the lesions most frequently seen. Hellier (1954) quotes the instance of one child who later developed severe acne having previously had infantile acne, but there are few other studies which document the outcome of the child with infantile acne.

6. *Tropical Acne*
When European and American soldiers have had to serve in the wet tropical climates of Malaya or Vietnam or elsewhere in the Far East, a particularly unpleasant type of acne has occurred. Those with extensive and severe acne seem to be more prone to this complication, but soldiers who were previously completely uninvolved may also develop tropical acne. It is one of the commonest causes of disability in these regions, and morbidity from this condition has been frequent amongst troops who fought in Vietnam. It is not entirely clear what factors predispose to this problem, but it is reasonable to assume that direct

climatic effects on the skin are involved. Those in air-conditioned offices do not develop this complication whereas the soldier on active duty in the same area does. Furthermore, it has been suggested that the wearing of heavy 'back packs' and the inability to bathe predispose to tropical acne. The back is particularly severely involved, although the face and chest may also be affected. Cystic lesions are common, and large inflamed papules are also seen. The lesions may spontaneously discharge, and as the condition is often extensive it may be extremely disabling. These patients spontaneously improve when they are removed to an air-conditioned and cooler atmosphere.

7. *Excoriated Acne*

This is sometimes colourfully called '*acné excoriée des jeunes filles*'. As men are amongst the sufferers from this complaint and as the '*filles*' are not always particularly '*jeunes*' there seems little justification for retention of this term. Frequently there are only very few typical acne lesions present, and the patients' complaints are clearly more than their physical appearance warrants. The lesions will be seen to be crusted and excoriated (*Fig.* 28) and often leave shallow pock-type scars. It is not uncommon for an anxious or obsessive youngster to pick at a few spots, but there are also patients where there seems to be a much more profound personality disorder, and in whom excoriated acne is particularly stubborn. Unfortunately, these patients continue to pick at their faces even after skilled psychiatric attention, although they may eventually seem to stop this practice for no very obvious reason.

8. *Papular Acne of Chin in Women*

This type of acne may not appear until the middle of the third decade or even later. As the name suggests, for some peculiar reason as yet without anatomical or physiological explanation, the chin is most frequently affected. Papules are the commonest lesions and they often look 'deep set' and indolent (*Fig.* 29). Premenstrual flare is characteristic and affected women complain that the papules become more prominent and tender 7–10 days before the period; a few pustules may erupt as well. There is some improvement on the day of the period or very shortly afterwards, but the deeper-set lesions may persist for some weeks. In addition, treatment is frequently ineffective and the condition can grumble on for some years. The clinical picture and history are sufficiently distinctive to merit separate consideration of this condition. Newman and Feldman (1954) describe this condition under the term 'adult premenstrual acne'. They stressed that lesions do not arise from comedones and described lesions on the side of the face as well as between the eyebrows. They suggested that this condition is associated with dysfunction of the corpus luteum.

9. *Senile Comedones*

These lesions (*Fig.* 30) are seen on the malar areas and periocularly in association with elastotic degeneration. Milia are often seen side by side with the comedones. They do not become inflamed and may represent pilosebaceous dilatation due to lack of connective tissue support.

10. *'Red Acne'*

There has been considerable confusion in the past concerning the relationship between acne and rosacea. The confusion has in part been caused by some patients with acne developing a background of erythema on the cheeks, chin and forehead (*Plate* 5A). The cause of this erythema may be damage to the subpapillary plexus from the inflammatory acne process. Some of these patients seem to recover completely, while others continue to develop inflammatory papules and then closely simulate true rosacea.

11. *Pomade Acne*

This term has been used to describe papular lesions of acne occurring on the forehead and temple particularly, but elsewhere on the face as well, that probably result from the continual use of oily hair dressings and grooming agents (Plewig, Fulton and Kligman, 1970). In a study of 735 Negro men, the lesions described were uniform closed comedones and small papules that were not often inflamed. The lesions could be induced by the application to the back of the various grooming agents, which seemed to differ in their degree of acneigenicity which was anyway weak. There are earlier reports from France of such acneiform lesions, due to the use of brilliantines and creams (Gougerot et al., 1945; Tzanck et al., 1945). It is possible that 'fringe or pop' acne described by Bowyer (1965) is a variant of pomade acne, rather than the result of shielding from the sun as suggested originally. In this latter variant, papules, pustules and comedones are found mostly beneath the fringe of hair that was fashionable when the entity was described, and to some extent still is. More recently Kligman and Mills (1972) have found that many oily materials will produce comedones when inuncted into the rabbit ear—including lanolin, petrolatum, vegetable oils, butyl stearate, lauryl alcohol and oleic acid.

12. *Scalp Pustules due to* Corynebacterium Acnes

This condition, described by Maibach (1967), is not really true acne, but as the author refers to it as the scalp analogue of acne and as it seems to be caused by *Corynebacterium acnes* and is helped by prolonged tetracyclines, it is best mentioned here. It is characterized by the eruption of discrete and turgid pustules over the whole scalp.

13. *Elastoplast Acne*

A peculiarly persistent type of acneiform folliculitis is sometimes seen under adhesive strapping that has been kept on for long periods. This seems most common after the misguided application of plaster strapping to the chest wall for fractured ribs.

14. *Hormonally Induced Acne*

Testosterone and other androgens can make pre-existing acne much worse, and can induce it for the first time in a eunuch.

All glucocorticoids can cause an acne type of rash. This is more common in young patients but is by no means confined to them. Cysts, very inflamed lesions and comedones are not seen in 'steroid' acne. Typically the eruption consists of a crop of uniform dark-red acneiform papules that appear suddenly and can disappear as suddenly after stopping treatment. Other signs of toxicity from glucocorticoids such as facial mooning, striae and hirsuties are usually present.

'*The Pill*.' Some varieties of contraceptive pill seem to help acne but others seem to provoke it or make it worse. Their action seems to depend on the relative concentrations of oestrogen- and progesterone-like compounds. The newer sequential pills seem marginally less troublesome in this respect.

15. *Other Types of Drug-induced Acne*

Acneiform drug eruptions are more often talked about than actually seen. The halogens and various halogenated compounds are classically described as causing an acneiform folliculitis. This is particularly true for the bromide-containing compounds although since the decline in the consumption of bromides this eruption is hardly ever seen. Bromides can, of course, cause vegetating and pyodermatous lesions. Iodinated drugs can also be acneigenic, although organically bound iodine seems to be innocent in this respect. Fluorides have not been incriminated, and neither have chlorides, although chlorinated naphthalene-containing oils are potent acneigens (*see below*). Other drugs, particularly phenytoin, trimethadione and isoniazid, have been cited as causes of drug-induced acne, but there is scanty evidence for a true association.

16. *Occupational Acne*

a. Oil Acne. Regrettably oil acne is a not uncommon industrial skin complaint. As Kligman and his group have shown, using the rabbit ear as a model, many oils and oily materials can be comedogenic. Most are weak acneigens. Whether they cause an acne-type eruption or not depends on the frequency and length of exposure to them. The oils that seem to be responsible for most cases of straightforward oil acne in industry are the insoluble cutting oils, and machinists are the most frequently affected workers. The lesions seen include numerous comedones, acne-type inflammatory papules and sometimes pustules. No age group is immune and the distribution of lesions depends on the area of contact. The traditional areas to be involved are the fronts of the thighs (and sometimes the groins and genitalia), the forearms and the face, as these are the areas of contact with oils (either directly or indirectly through oil-soaked overalls). However, any hairy area can be affected. Cysts are not usually seen. The oil acne may be accompanied by oil melanosis or even by oil keratoses (Schwartz et al., 1947). Crude petroleum has been responsible for oil acne in oilfield workers and in oil refineries. Coal tar and tar distillates can cause similar problems for tar distillers, roadmakers and others who work with these products, including makers of insulating materials and labourers using creosote.

b. Chloracne. This subject has been comprehensively reviewed by Crow (1970). Herxheimer (1899) was the first to describe an acneiform eruption occurring on the face and arms of workers exposed to chlorine gas produced electrolytically. He believed that chlorine was the cause, but later it was realized that chlorinated aromatic hydrocarbons were responsible. The various compounds that have been incriminated include the chlornaphthalenes, the chlorbiphenyls, the chlorphenols and the chlorbenzols.

These chlorinated compounds are potent acneigens and acne lesions may start to appear as little as 1 month after exposure. The workers exposed to these chemicals are usually employed making electrical insulating materials or they may be in the chemical industry. Jones and Alden (1936) described the lesions occurring with chlorinated hydrocarbons as starting on the face, round the angles of the jaws, or over the malar areas and spreading to the sides of the face and the back of the neck and later to the arms (*Fig.* 31). The lesions were comedones, papules, pustules and small cysts, and a distinguishing feature of this type of acne was its itchiness.

A most useful contribution to this subject was that of Shelley and Kligman (1957). They painted various chlornaphthalenes on to volunteers, and found that 50 per cent penta- and hexachlornaphthalenes (Halowax 1014) in mineral oil invariably led to the production of acne in 31 subjects in all areas to which they were applied. Not only was the material acneigenic in areas of application, but also in distant sites due to the subjects inadvertently spreading the compounds manually. Comedones started to appear within 4–6 weeks. Unfortunately, lesions continued to develop after stopping application at 2 months, and reached a zenith at 4 months. Inflammatory acne indistinguishable from acne conglobata was produced in all subjects. The lesions produced were monitored histologically. At first large keratin-filled sacs were produced and later the sebaceous glands began to atrophy and disappear. This was followed by intrafollicular and perifollicular inflammation with eventual follicular rupture and abscess formation. Thus, in contrast to ordinary acne, abscess formation stems from the comedo.

Crow (1970) has drawn attention to a report from Japan (Katsuki et al., 1969) in which there was accidental contamination of a cooking oil by tetrachlorbiphenyl, which was used as a heat-exchange medium. The contamination amounted to 2000 p.p.m. of the chlorbiphenyl. Approximately 5 or 6 g of these materials were consumed by these patients in 5 or 6 months. Swelling of the meibomian glands with discharge of a cheese-like material was an early physical sign. Comedones and small cysts were mostly present but papules and pustules also occurred in some. A widespread follicular hyperkeratosis was also noted in these patients, and this has been noted previously in association with chloracne (Crow, 1970).

17. *Acne Necrotica*

This is usually subdivided into acne necrotica varioliformis and acne necrotica miliaris. The first form is characterized, as its name suggests, by lesions leaving large varioliform scars, while the second is so named because there are very many smaller lesions. They are probably variants of the same disorder. Both types are relatively uncommon though the miliary variety is the more often encountered. Clinically the typical lesion, both large and small, is a conical brownish-red papule, topped by a black adherent crust. The papules are mostly distributed on the forehead, temple and scalp. The disorder may persist for some years and there is no specific treatment. The cause of acne necrotica is unknown and whether it is related to ordinary acne or not is uncertain. Some suggest that these lesions represent no more than enthusiastic excoriation.

DIFFERENTIAL DIAGNOSIS

1. The occasional difficulty in distinguishing the condition from rosacea is discussed elsewhere (p. 38) but in general the lack of persistent erythema, telangiectasia or symmetry and the presence of comedones and cysts distinguish acne from rosacea.

2. Perioral dermatitis is sometimes mistaken for acne, but the uniformity of the small papules and the lack of other lesions distinguish perioral dermatitis.

3. Acneiform papules are seen in acne agminata but these lesions are brownish-red and granulomatous-looking and should not be confused with true acne papules.

4. Papulonecrotic tuberculide is a follicular process and lesions may be seen on the cheeks and forehead. The presence of lesions elsewhere and the central necrosis and crusting distinguish this uncommon condition.

5. An acneiform rash is sometimes seen in secondary syphilis. The lesions are often in the nasolabial grooves and have a 'moist' appearance. They are often in a patterned arrangement. The history and coexisting manifestations of the condition should also help distinguish this from acne.

6. Occasionally plane warts, mollusca contagiosa, milia and sarcoid lesions are also mistaken for acne.

INFLUENCE OF DIET ON ACNE

Traditionally certain foods are supposed to make acne worse. Chocolate, nuts, fats and fried foods, pork and carbohydrate foodstuffs are amongst those blamed for relapses and exacerbations. As pointed out by Fulton et al. (1969), all the 'forbidden foods' have one thing in common—they are delicious and delectable to the adolescent taste. A cynic could be forgiven for believing that some of the austere diets proposed for acne were designed more to punish the patient than to influence his acne.

In the writer's experience most patients find no special relationship between any particular food and the development of new acne lesions or the worsening of old ones. Admittedly, some state with a suspicious vehemence that milk or chocolate or some other foodstuff makes their acne worse. It is impossible to evaluate these claims as they are uncontrolled observations by unskilled observers who are, in addition, emotionally involved. On delving it seems that, as in rosacea, folklore is at the root of the idea of a connection between diet and acne. Unfortunately it has often been uncritically perpetuated by physicians, who are responsible for implanting the idea of a food relationship in some patients. Undoubtedly body fat is influenced by diet, and it is possible that sebum can occasionally also be affected, but the sebaceous glands do not 'excrete' lipids. Thus, Lipkin et al. (1968) infused radioactively labelled eriolein, palmitate, cholesterol and cholesterol esters into a skin flap in dogs. Less than 1 per cent was recovered from the epidermis or sebaceous glands.

Apparently, there is one way in which sebaceous secretion can be influenced dietetically and that is by total starvation! Pochi et al. (1970) found that the total amount of sebum secreted by 11 obese patients who were being therapeutically starved fell by an average of 40 per cent. In addition, sebum was found to change in composition in these and other starved patients. There was no change in the amount of squalene secreted, but the amounts of triglyceride, fatty acids, wax esters, cholesterol and cholesterol esters fell. They also suggest that less drastic alterations of calorie intake may influence the composition of sebum. Clearly this is a challenging contribution that should be followed up.

MacDonald (1968) gave chocolate to 29 adolescents for 5 days and found that this increased the cholesterol content of the surface lipids while the triglyceride in the surface lipids diminished in men but not in women. He also claimed that both starch and sucrose supplements caused some increase in the straight-chain C16 mono-unsaturated fatty acid, but only starch increased the saturated C16 acid. Fulton et al. (1969), in a delightfully iconoclastic paper, removed chocolate from the villain's role in the acne drama. They fed either an enriched chocolate bar or a control bar (identical in appearance and similar in taste but without any chocolate) to 65 acne subjects. This was a cross-over blind study, the bars being fed 1 daily for 4 weeks with a 3-week rest period between 'treatments'. Assessments were made by counting lesions at weekly intervals. With the chocolate bar 46 subjects were unchanged, 10 were better and 9 worse, while after taking the control bar 53 were unchanged, 5 were better and 7 worse. In addition, 5 healthy subjects ate 2 enriched chocolate bars per day for 1 month without any apparent significant effect on the quantity or composition of the sebum secreted. Similar conclusions had been reached by Grant and Anderson in 1965 by feeding chocolate to 8 subjects.

ACNE AND PSYCHE

Luckily we are moving out of the era when every disease with an obscure cause was laid at the feet of Freud. The literature is replete with reference to various disturbances of the psyche in patients with acne.

However, when these reports are examined few stand up to critical evaluation. Kenyon (1966) reviewed the subject and from his own investigations concluded that acne is not primarily a psychogenic condition. However, Kenyon added that he thought that this skin condition could be exacerbated as the result of emotional stress and that there is a marked tendency for secondary psychological effects to take the form of social isolation. Lucas (1961) in a controlled study on students, in whom Maudsley personality inventories were used, found no especial tendency to neuroticism or extroversion in the group with acne. Similarly there were no more psychological symptoms in the acne sufferers than in the control students. Nonetheless, acne patients are frequently quite depressed because of disfigurement caused by acne. Young women are frequently told that their acne will improve when they marry or when they have a child. This again seems to be uncritical advice and part of dermatological folklore. Ratzer in 1964 found no basis for believing that marriage had any substantial effect, though she found that childbirth did produce some improvement.

HISTOPATHOLOGY

The histopathology of acne has been sadly neglected and neither Pinkus and Mehregan (1969) nor Lever and Lever (1975) discuss the subject in detail. Acne is essentially a follicular process and the changes seen will, to some extent, depend on the type of lesion biopsied and its stage of development.

Comedones
Both 'open' and 'closed' comedones are dilated hair follicles containing keratinous debris and inspissated sebum. Lynch (1940) pointed out that there is frequently parakeratotic horn within the comedo. In addition, Gram-positive rods and coccal forms can be found in the follicle. Kligman et al. (1970) have found that follicles in which a comedo has been experimentally induced show a curious irregular epithelial hypertrophy. This change, that has also been observed by Wilson-Jones and Marks (1973, unpublished observations), is almost naevoid in its appearance and is at the moment without explanation (*Fig.* 32).

Papules
These lesions appear to be the result of a folliculitis or a perifolliculitis. Strauss and Kligman (1960) demonstrated that a breach in follicular epithelium allows the escape of follicular contents into the perifollicular dermis. Early inflammatory lesions may show only a slight cellular infiltrate around the area of follicular damage composed mainly of polymorphs and lymphocytes. Older lesions show much more follicular disruption and more granulomatous inflammation. Giant cells and large histiocytes are sometimes seen especially around keratinous debris and follicular remnants. A variable amount of scarring is seen in the upper and mid dermis.

Pustules
Pustules are basically tiny abscesses. They contain masses of polymorphs and cellular debris and are often based on a closed comedo blocked by keratinous debris. Strauss and Kligman (1960) thought that pustules might also result from rupture of closed comedones, and that on occasions there may be a true bacterial impetigo of the follicle.

Cysts
These are best called 'pseudocysts' as there is no epithelial lining and they are in reality 'cold abscesses'. Histologically there is an extensive

area in the dermis occupied by inflammatory cell infiltrate and cellular debris. The infiltrate is surrounded by a zone of granulation tissue and a variable amount of fibrosis. Cells of all types are seen in the area of infiltration. Polymorphs are prominent in places, while large histiocytes and foreign-body-type giant cells are seen focally. Elsewhere lymphocytes and histiocytes are seen and plasma cells may be particularly prominent, especially if the biopsy is from the back of the neck (*Fig.* 33).

Acne Pits and Pock Marks

Strauss and Kligman (1956) have shown that pits are often unexpectedly tortuous and filled with keratinous debris. The follicular epithelium may be markedly hypertrophied and irregular, and vellus hair regrowth may be seen in the pit.

Watson (1959) claimed that pock marks arose from the destruction of the tissue bridges and grooves to complex 'polyporous follicles'.

General Considerations

The follicular disruption and related inflammation are characteristic for acne. The lack of oedema and of telangiectasia, the absence of prominent elastotic degeneration and of upper dermal disorganization help distinguish acne from rosacea.

If presented with an acne biopsy showing predominantly granulomatous inflammation, accurate histological diagnosis may be very difficult. Nevertheless, the presence of large numbers of polymorphs interposed in the inflamed areas together with the presence of follicular debris is helpful in reaching the right conclusion.

AETIOLOGY AND PATHOGENESIS

Much work has been done in an attempt to understand the mechanisms of acneigenesis. Attention has been paid in particular to the factors controlling sebaceous gland secretion and to the bacteriology of acne. In the discussion of the aetiology of acne that follows, attention will be focussed on: 'The comedo and the hair follicles'; 'The control of secretion of sebum'; and 'The bacteriology of acne'.

The Comedo and the Hair Follicle

It is often assumed (probably correctly) that the formation of the comedo is an essential step in the pathogenesis of acne. The concept of Strauss and Kligman (1960) was that the visible blackhead (the open comedo) is less harmful than the 'explosion' of the 'time bomb' of the closed follicle with the obstructed narrow neck. The factors that might be concerned in comedo formation and follicular obstruction are as follows:

a. Anatomical abnormality of follicular opening.

b. Increased viscosity of sebum.

c. Decreased drainage of follicle by underdeveloped hair.

d. Weak arrectores pilorum muscles allowing stagnation of sebum.

In fact, insufficient experimental work has been done to investigate adequately these possibilities. One extremely interesting piece of work was that of Van Scott and MacCardle (1956). These workers found that the earliest change of acne was hyperkeratinization of the excretory duct of the sebaceous gland which results in the deposition of a keratinous plug in the follicular neck. However, Vasarinsh (1969) could not detect any abnormality of keratinization of sebaceous ducts in serial sections from acne biopsies and found that rupture of acne cyst walls can take place in follicles with patent ostia. Attention seems to have riveted on the cause of the inflammatory reaction rather than on the possibility of an underlying follicular abnormality. The characteristic anatomical distribution of acne might also suggest that structural factors in the follicle are important. Acne of the scalp and of areas where there is a strong beard growth is uncommon. Many of the early writers on acne made much of this particular point, suggesting that where sebum could drain away by the 'wick action' of the hair, follicular obstruction was unlikely to occur. Grant (1957) studied the relation between the severity of acne and the incidence of follicles with 'succeeding hairs' and thought that 'the factor which precipitates comedo formation in acne vulgaris is the absence of an effective hair'. In addition, those sites that are affected are those possessing follicles with prominent sebaceous glands. Oil acne in some way produces follicular irritation, hyperkeratosis and comedo formation and finally proper acne, and it has also been suggested that steroid acne also results from abnormal follicular keratinization.

The Control of Secretion of Sebum

1. The following facts first suggested a relationship between the male sex hormones on the one hand and sebum secretion on the other:

i. Acne starts at puberty and reaches its maximum incidence in adolescence (at age 16 according to Munro-Ashman, 1963).

ii. Acne does not occur in eunuchs until androgenic substances are administered.

iii. Acne occurs as part of the virilizing syndromes and Cushing's syndrome.

iv. Acne occurs after the administration of androgenic substances to women (Barsone and Reisnes, 1971).

2. In statistical terms acne patients secrete more sebum than a matched control group. However, this does not necessarily apply to the individual. Every clinician has seen the greasy-skinned patient without

acne. Cunliffe and Shuster (1969) found that the severity of acne was related to the degree of seborrhoea and they were of the opinion that 'Acne cannot develop without an increased rate of sebum excretion. . .'. Interestingly they found that when clinical acne regressed the seborrhoea persisted. Pochi and Strauss (1964) found an overall increase in the rate of sebum excretion in acne patients compared to controls, but no direct correlation, and similar findings were reported by Powell and Beveridge (1970).

It should be added here that Plewig (1974) found using tritiated thymidine and autoradiography and planimetry that the increased sebum secretion of acne is due to increased sebaceous gland cell proliferation and a concomitant increase in sebaceous gland size.

3. The following conclusions have been reached mainly from animal experiments, and although they have mostly been verified in man this is not true in every instance.

 a. Androgens increase the amount of sebum excreted.

 b. Androgens increase the size of sebaceous glands in the castrated animal.

 c. Hypophysectomy prevents full expression of this androgen effect on sebaceous glands.

 d. Oestrogens decrease the amount of sebum excreted (Jarrett, 1955), and also decrease the size of sebaceous glands. Ebling (1954) thought that this might be due to a direct effect on the sebaceous gland, rather than an indirect effect acting via the pituitary.

The results were interpreted as indicating that oestrogens affect the holocrine secretion of the sebaceous gland and epidermal keratinization and that these actions were independent of any possible influence on the mitotic rates. However, Strauss et al. (1962) found no suppression of sebum when oestrogen was administered in physiological doses, and suggested that any suppressive action was due to a pharmacological suppression of the pituitary–ovarian axis.

To add to the confusion Pochi et al. (1965) found that patients with acne demonstrated increased plasma 17-beta oestradiol and oestrone, but not testosterone when compared to controls.

 e. The action of progesterone is uncertain. Strauss and Kligman (1961) gave progesterone in 'physiological amounts' to 8 prepubertal men and women, 11 postpubertal men and women and 3 aged females. They did not see any significant change in sebaceous gland size or function. In addition, they could not detect any fluctuation in sebum production in different phases of the menstrual cycle. However, progesterone is known to have some androgenic effects experimentally in rats (Greene et al., 1939; Haskin et al., 1953).

4. Glucocorticoids appear to have very little effect on sebaceous gland function. Contrary to expectation (in view of steroid acne), glucocorticoids do not have any androgenic activity as far as sebaceous glands are concerned. In fact, experimental evidence has shown the reverse. Pochi and Strauss (1967) administered prednisone to 7 normal men, 12 normal women and 8 castrated men, and found that sebum secretion, measured gravimetrically, was depressed in the castrated male group, although it had no effect on the normal males. This suggested to them the possibility that normally in these two groups sebaceous secretion was under the control of adrenocortical androgens.

5. Pituitary hormones themselves might have some sebaceous gland activity and the existence of a 'sebotrophin' has been suggested. However, normal levels of growth hormone have been found in patients with acne (Strafford et al., 1969). Shuster's group has given serious consideration to the possibility of alpha-MSH playing a role in influencing the rate of sebum secretion (Goolamali et al., 1973). However, their view at the time of writing is that this peptide is probably not involved.

6. The viscosity of sebum is normal in acne patients compared to matched controls (Burton, 1970) and the composition of sebum in acne patients appears identical to that in controls.

7. An interesting approach to sebaceous gland function has been that of a Glasgow group who have made a histochemical study of the presence and activity of steroid dehydrogenases in the sebaceous glands from various sites and age groups. It was originally claimed that 3-alpha, 3-beta, 11-beta, 16-beta and 17-beta hydroxysteroid dehydrogenases were detectable in sebaceous glands from the upper back, face and presternal region, but not in those from the limbs, perineal, perivulval or penile skin (Baillie et al., 1966), and that activity was greatest in young adult life. However, subsequent investigation found a more anatomically uniform distribution of steroid dehydrogenase activity (Calman et al., 1970). The significance of the presence of these enzymes is uncertain. They may only be a reflection of the importance of androgen metabolism for these structures.

8. Sebum contains cholesterol, cholesterol esters, triglycerides, waxes, fatty acids and squalene (Downing et al., 1969). Practically all the constituents of sebum have been shown to be capable of inducing comedones in the rabbit-ear model (Kligman et al., 1970). However, the biological importance of a particular fraction in the production of comedones depends on its relative comedogenicity and its concentration in the sebum. Thus, squalene is a potent comedo producer, but is only present in concentrations of up to 10 per cent, and so is relatively unimportant *in vivo* in the production of comedones. The most important comedogenic components of sebum are the triglycerides and the fatty

acids. The latter are strongly comedogenic but variable in amount. Kligman and his co-workers conclude that the higher even-numbered saturated and mono-unsaturated fatty acids ($C16 : 0$, $C16 : 1$, $C18 : 0$, $C18 : 1$) mainly account for the comedogenicity of sebum, and constitute about 75 per cent of the total free fatty acid content.

Kellum and Strangfeld (1972) found a greater concentration of a fatty acid by gas liquid chromotography in acne patients. This was later identified (Krakow et al., 1973) as octa-deca-5,8-dienoic acid.

9. It has frequently been suggested that inflamed lesions in acne are caused by the passage of sebum through the follicular wall and into the dermis (the irritant constituents of sebum being the fatty acids released from the triglycerides by bacterial hydrolysis—*see below*).

Nicolaides and Wells (1957) examined sebaceous material from lesions of steatocystoma multiplex and found no free fatty acids. They also found that hydrolysis of triglycerides took place shortly after delivery of sebum on to the surface and that there was a non-specific esterase activity that could be responsible for the lipolysis, where the sebum enters the hair canal. Kellum (1967) examined sebaceous glands isolated from the scalp and extracted lipids from this tissue and then analysed them by thin-layer chromatography. Only squalene wax esters and triglycerides were found. Thus, it seems that fatty acids are not found in freshly formed sebum, but only arise later when released on to the skin surface by lipolysis of the triglycerides.

Strauss and Pochi (1965) injected intracutaneously small quantities of sebum, the various constituents of sebum, suspensions of comedones and sebum from which the fatty acids had been removed into the backs of 51 subjects. Biopsies were taken of the test sites. It was found that whole sebum and the fatty acid fraction produced equally severe inflammatory reactions, characterized by follicular disruption and a marked lymphocytic infiltrate. Sebum without fatty acids, and the other constituents of sebum, did not induce marked inflammatory reactions, when injected. When comedo suspensions from which the fatty acids had been removed were injected, a giant cell reaction was often produced. Furthermore, the reaction of acne patients was not different in any way from that of the other subjects, and sebum from acne patients did not cause any greater reaction than sebum from normal subjects. Kellum (1968) found that the most irritant fatty acids were in the C8–C14 range when these compounds were applied under occlusive dressings. He believed that the reaction produced by these fatty acids in the test he devised was due partly to their irritant properties and partly to their good percutaneous absorption.

It seems then that fatty acids may be both comedogenic and irritant but that different chain lengths are concerned in these two pathogenic actions. One point not satisfactorily answered experimentally is the predominantly polymorphonuclear inflammatory response seen in the disease, as against the mainly lymphocytic reaction noted in artificially induced lesions.

10. Powell and Beveridge (1970) have drawn attention to the wax ester constituent of sebum as they have found that these substances are markedly lower in concentration in the sebum of young men without acne as compared to those with acne. In addition, the wax esters fall and the triglycerides increase during remission induced by tetracycline (Beveridge and Powell, 1969), and after the application of 2-naphthol peeling paste (Powell, 1970). The significance of this unexpected correlation of 'acne activity' with the wax ester content of sebum remains unexplained for the moment.

The Bacteriology of Acne

Because of the presence of pustules, the pus-like contents of cystic lesions and the good response of acne to certain antibiotics, there would seem to be good reason for supposing bacterial infection plays an important part in the disease. However, it is now established beyond all reasonable doubt that acne is not caused by pathogenic bacteria in the same sense that boils or impetigo are. Early reports in which *Staphylococcus aureus* or other pathogenic bacteria were thought to be important can be discounted. An apt statement in this regard is that of Shehadeh and Kligman (1963) who say: 'The student wishing to learn about the kinds of organisms in acne lesions must be firmly advised not to consult the literature. It is a bramble thicket which will scratch rather than supply the mind. In confusion, contradiction and in sheer wealth of error, it is a classic in dermatomythology.' The subject has been critically reviewed by Rosenberg (1969). Unna in 1896 described rod-shaped bacteria in acne lesions, and in 1897 Sabouraud cultured the bacillus now called *Corynebacterium acnes*. This organism is today recognized as part of the normal skin flora and known to be micro-aerophilic or anaerobic. In 1961 Smith and Waterworth reported that they could only find *Staphylococcus albus* and *C. acnes* in 67 lesions of acne from 39 patients, and no differences were detected in the various types of lesion. In 1963 Shehadeh and Kligman examined the lesions from 100 patients and concluded that *C. acnes* and *Staph. albus* were the only significant micro-organisms isolated, and that they existed as a 'stable biad'. Marples and Izumi (1970) bacteriologically examined 107 small acne pustules from 27 patients. They found the same two micro-organisms predominating. In 2 patients they isolated *Enterobacter aeorgenes* and it was thought that these two patients could be examples of the Gram-negative folliculitis seen occasionally (Fulton et al., 1968; and *see below*).

In 8 patients lipophilic diphtheroids were found, but not in great numbers. *C. acnes* and the Gram-positive cocci occurred together in half the pustules, and of these *C. acnes* dominated in 27, the Gram-positive cocci dominated in 16, while equal numbers were recorded in 7. The staphylococci were classified according to the Baird-Parker scheme and a greater number of the SII strain was found compared to the normal facial flora. The same authors also looked at the acne comedo bacteriologically (Izumi et al., 1970), and found that in 45 comedones examined (both 'open' and 'closed'), *C. acnes* and Gram-positive cocci were present in every case. Interestingly SII cocci were again dominant, but they found a higher density of *C. acnes* in closed comedones.

Thus, the dominant flora of acne ('the stable biad') consists of the same two micro-organisms normally found on the face and it seems that they are not 'prime movers' in the acne process. The important role that has been assigned to *C. acnes* as a supplier of esterases, with which the triglycerides are split, still has the status of a hypothesis and is unsupported by solid evidence. Some have suggested that the yeast-like micro-organism often found in follicles—the *Pityrosporon ovale*—is implicated in the pathogenesis of acne. However, the evidence for this is also slim. Although lipase activity has been detected in these organisms (Marples et al., 1972) it should also be mentioned that other bacterial enzymes may be important in the production of acne lesions. For example, *C. acnes* has been found to produce hyaluronidase (Puhvel and Reisner, 1972).

Prolonged antibacterial treatment for acne, including the use of antibacterial soaps and systemic antibiotics, can apparently cause 'superinfection' with Gram-negative bacteria resulting in crops of pustules. Fulton et al. (1968) describe 6 such patients. Not only were the Gram-negative rods persistently recovered from pustules on the face, but they were also found in the nares. Histologically these lesions differed from ordinary acne pustules in having no comedonal 'core'.

Kellum and Strangfeld (1970) wondered whether *C. acnes* made irritant fatty acids, either as extracellular metabolic products or as structural fatty acids liberated after bacterial death. They found no qualitative or quantitative differences in the fatty acids liberated from *C. acnes* derived from acne patients and controls, and concluded that irritant fatty acids are not derived from *C. acnes*. Other work by the same group (Kellum et al., 1970) suggests that *C. acnes*, rather than *Staphylococcus epidermidis*, is important in the hydrolysis of triglyceride, and that distinctive strains of *C. acnes* are involved. Increased levels of antibody to *C. acnes* (but not to *Staph. epidermidis*) have been found in the sera of patients with papulopustular and cystic acne compared to normal controls (Puhvel et al., 1964, 1965).

Summary

A convenient working hypothesis for the production of acne lesions is as follows.

Increased androgenic influence (or perhaps increased end-organ responsiveness) produces sebaceous gland hyperplasia and seborrhoea. Comedo formation results from the seborrhoea and perhaps from an abnormality of keratinization at the follicular mouth. Follicular damage is induced mainly in those follicles with large sebaceous glands and only weak hair growth and which have small blocked ostia (sebaceous follicles). Fatty acids are liberated by hydrolysis from triglycerides in sebum with bacterial esterases liberated from *C. acnes* high in the follicles (perhaps *Staph. epidermidis* contributes to the lipolysis). The fatty acids diffuse through intact (or perhaps through ruptured) follicular walls and cause inflammation and follicular disruption. Liberated keratin from the injured follicles evokes a granulomatous response in the dermis.

TREATMENT

The tendency for acne to improve and the fluctuating remittent course bedevil attempts at assessing the efficiency of any form of treatment. In addition the difficulty in quantitating changes in the condition should make one wary when assessing reports of the efficacy of new therapeutic agents.

Topical Treatments

In general, topical treatments are messy and only marginally helpful. They are, however, sometimes useful in superficial acne, and may be all that is required for this mild type of disease.

Desquamative Agents

These are supposed to work by helping to unblock the follicles, but it is difficult to imagine that this can be their only mode of action in every case.

Sulphur in various concentrations (2–12 per cent) is still one of the most widely prescribed agents in this category. A popular preparation suitable for most is 5 per cent sulphur in calamine lotion. Hardier skins can tolerate 9 per cent or even 12 per cent concentrations of sulphur. Sulphurated potash is another preparation that is often used. There is virtually no information as to why sulphur is irritant and an effective peeling agent. Its effectiveness has actually been questioned recently. Mills and Kligman (1972) found sulphur comedogenic in the rabbit ear and suggested that it could be harmful in treatment. Its action might be related to that of the sulphides and thioglycolates which work by rupturing the disulphide linkage in keratin by forming hydrogen sulphide. Some individuals cannot tolerate sulphur preparations even in concentrations as low as 1 or 2 per cent and develop a primary irritant dermatitis. The patients most likely to react in this way are those with fair hair and blue eyes, while those with red hair and pink complexions are even more at risk.

Resorcin and *beta-naphthol* (2-naphthol) are other active ingredients of some peeling preparations, though they are infrequently used now. The reason for their effectiveness is uncertain, but recently Powell (1970) demonstrated a considerable drop in the rate of sebum secretion from the forehead of young men whose acne had been treated by 2-naphthol (beta-naphthol) peeling paste elsewhere on the body. Concomitant with the drop in the rate of secretion was a fall in the wax ester content of the sebum. Presumably, the reason for the effect 'at a distance' must result from the systemic absorption of 2-naphthol or a derivative from the site of its application.

Benzoyl peroxide in concentrations of up to 10 per cent is available with and without sulphur and hydroxyquinoline in various proprietary preparations. Its use was described and recommended by Pace (1965) and it seems moderately successful on occasions for superficial acne. It is a powerful oxidizing agent and presumably its keratolytic effect depends on this property. As with sulphur, some individuals cannot tolerate the primary irritation it causes. In addition, it can produce a true allergic contact dermatitis. It may also have an antibacterial effect.

Abrasive agents must be included in this group. They contain silica particles of graded size and are designed to promote follicular drainage by producing a mild desquamation.

Retinoic acid has been used topically in acne (Kligman et al., 1969) and it certainly seems to produce a brisk inflammatory reaction with desquamation. Its mode of action is uncertain but presumably is related to the profound effect that vitamin A has on the granular layer. Other authors have found retinoic acid helpful in topical preparations.

Antibacterial Preparations

These are employed in the hope that they will reduce the local flora sufficiently to inhibit their supposed role in the lipolysis of the triglycerides of sebum, and thus prevent the liberation of fatty acids. It should be emphasized that in general these agents are not very effective either at significantly decreasing the flora or improving the skin. They are in addition often expensive and may be sensitizing.

Hexachlorophene as a detergent emulsion is often prescribed for use instead of soap but is of unproven value, and could be harmful because of absorption.

Hydroxyquinolines are used in some proprietary preparations in combination with benzoyl peroxide or other compounds.

Antibiotics including neomycin, the tetracyclines and erythromycin have been used, and early suggestions are that they are quite successful on occasions—especially erythromycin. Sulphacetamide in combination with sulphur has also been recommended by Olansky (1967). He claimed 98 per cent excellent or good results, without adverse effects in 459 patients over a 2-year period! This study was uncontrolled and the way assessments were made was unstated. Apart from these considerations topical sulphonamides tend to produce sensitization and are best avoided.

Topical Corticosteroids

These are present in a number of proprietary preparations that are widely used. Both hydrocortisone and the more topically potent corticosteroids have been employed. The reasoning behind their use presumably is that as they are non-specific anti-inflammatory agents, they should reduce the inflammation seen in acne. However, they seem curiously inactive in this respect. Their failure may be due to the difficulty in penetrating to a sufficient depth in high enough concentration effectively to reduce the inflammation. However, they are helpful when employed intralesionally for cysts and scars (*see below*).

Systemic Treatments

Antibiotics and Sulphonamides

Virtually all have been recommended at some time, but the tetracyclines are most widely used, while erythromycin and the sulphonamides are still employed by some.

Tetracyclines. Although these compounds have been used for approximately 20 years in the treatment of acne, there is still controversy concerning their effectiveness and mode of action. There is a huge literature in which their use is described. Unfortunately, few of these investigations were designed to produce an unbiased answer and the few well-constructed trials have yielded conflicting results. Crounse (1965) and Fry and Ramsay (1966) did not find any beneficial action of tetracycline compared to a placebo, and the first author pointed out the very marked placebo response seen in his patients and in other investigations. Similarly Smith et al. (1962) found no benefit from administration of tetracyclines over the placebo-treated group. The other view has been represented by the thoughtful contributions of Savin and Turner (1966) and Lane and Williamson (1969). The first authors found a 78 per cent effectiveness for a tetracycline–novobiocin combination compared to improvement in 47 per cent of the placebo-treated group. Savin and Turner also suggested that it was necessary to use local therapy at the same time as antibiotic to demonstrate a significant response. Lane and Williamson investigated 51 patients in a double-blind trial in which tetracycline 250 mg twice daily was compared with a placebo. They assessed their patients clinically and photographically and concluded that 75 per cent of the treated group responded compared with a 33 per cent placebo response at 3 months. Cunliffe et al. (1973) found a satisfactory clinical response to tetracycline with a serum level of 1·98 ng/ml. They found a decreased concentration of fatty acids in the skin surface lipids but no decrease in bacterial flora accompanied the clinical response.

A very serious objection to obtaining any sort of coherent picture from the published results of trials is the lack of any uniformity and comparability in the various investigations.

Not only have different antibiotics been used including such variations on the tetracycline molecule as oxytetracycline, methacycline, demethylchlortetracycline or doxycycline, but also antibiotic combinations such as the tetracycline novobiocin mixture used by Savin and Turner (1966). In addition, different doses of the drugs have been used for different periods of time, and varying methods of assessment have been used. Many trials have used a 'lesion-counting method' (for example, the study of doxycycline by Plewig, Petrozzi and Berendes, 1970). Others have used a photographic method or some other means of clinical assessment. Furthermore, experimental design has varied from the double-blind cross-over study to the straight anecdotal reporting of the effect of treatment on a group of patients. Finally, the dermatologist's whim seems to have governed whether local treatments are used at the same time or not.

Notwithstanding all these issues, the balance of informed opinion is that the tetracyclines are effective in acne. A regime often prescribed is oxytetracycline (or tetracycline) 250 mg three times daily for the first week followed by a reduction in dose to 250 mg twice daily for 3 weeks. At 4 weeks the dose is adjusted to the smallest that will control the appearance of new lesions which may be as small as 250 mg on alternate days. Variability in absorption of the drug and in its delivery to the skin must be borne in mind. The tetracyclines should be taken before meals, as it has been suggested that they can chelate with calcium in foodstuffs and avoid absorption. The tetracyclines vary in their effectiveness and it has been suggested by Marples and Kligman (1971) that they vary in their delivery to the skin, and that dosages based on blood levels take no account of metabolical degradation after the drug enters epithelial cells.

Side-effects of tetracyclines: These are remarkably few and far between. The greatest theoretical danger is overwhelming superinfection of the bowel with either *Candida* or a resistant staphylococcus. Luckily, this appears to be extremely uncommon. Minor diarrhoea is occasionally seen, presumably due to minor alterations in gut flora or direct irritation of the bowel wall.

Marples et al. (1969) have shown that continuous tetracycline therapy leads to a decrease in the number of *C. acnes* in the nostrils and a concomitant increase in the numbers of enterobacteria recovered. There was, at the same time, a drop in the numbers of *Staph. aureus*, but an increase in the population of *Staph. epidermidis*. The increasing population of Gram-negative bacteria may be hazardous. It certainly seems to lead to the formation of acneiform pustules on occasions (*see above*). In addition Weary et al. (1969) described a young woman in whom tetracycline seemed to provoke an acneiform rash that appeared to be due to overgrowth of *Pityrosporon orbiculare*. Power (1970) documented a young man who became ill while on tetracycline and a corticosteroid, and from whose acne lesions a *Proteus* species was cultured. Certainly the possibility of clinical sequelae resulting from the altered ecological situation should be remembered. Tetracycline should not, of course, be administered to a pregnant woman because of the danger of discoloration and dystrophy of the teeth of the infant.

A fixed drug eruption is recorded as a result of tetracycline and should not be forgotten. Phototoxicity with a severe sunburn type of reaction is particularly common in demethyl-chlortetracycline and it is probably wiser not to prescribe this drug for acne patients for this reason.

Other Antibiotics. Erythromycin is probably the most frequently prescribed antibiotic next to tetracycline but its use is inadequately documented. Robinson (1964) describes erythromycin stearate as a valuable supplement in the treatment of acne but there does not appear to be a critically constructed trial in which its use has been properly investigated. It seems moderately safe, though the same cautions apply with regard to 'superinfection' as with the tetracyclines.

Virtually every antibiotic has been used at some time, including novobiocin, streptomycin and clindamycin but no convincing advantage has been detected over the tetracyclines.

Sulphonamides. These have often been recommended, for example by Andrews (1965) and Robinson (1964). Their use would appear to be potentially hazardous and without much justification as less toxic chemotherapeutic agents are available.

Mode of Action of Antibiotics. The response of acne to antibiotics appears mysterious for the following reasons:

  a. Only normal bacterial flora is recoverable from acne lesions.
  b. Small 'suboptimal' doses are often all that are required.
  c. Improvement takes place only after 2–4 weeks of treatment. Relapse, if it takes place, occurs after approximately 2 weeks.

d. Penicillin appears clinically ineffective although the flora is sensitive to it.

Freinkel (1969) believes that all the observed facts are compatible with an antibiotic action of the tetracyclines on the normal skin flora and a consequent reduction in bacterial lipolysis and fatty acid production. Certainly, reduction in normal bacterial flora after tetracycline therapy has been demonstrated (Goltz and Kjartansson, 1966), and a fall in fatty acid concentration in sebum during treatment has also been found (Freinkel et al., 1965).

Nonetheless, Beveridge and Powell (1969) found that tetracycline treatment produced a drop in the wax content of sebum of patients with acne and others have also expressed reservations as to the mode of action of tetracyclines (Marks and Davies, 1969). Certainly the tetracyclines are known to have profound biological effects besides their antibiotic actions, and it may be that these are more important in acne. It is of interest in this respect that the tetracyclines have been shown to inhibit lipase activity *in vitro* independently of their antibiotic action (Shalita and Wheatley, 1970).

Corticosteroids

It is paradoxically true that systemic steroids are sometimes of use in acne. It is only when the acne is very inflamed, extensive and severe that the use of steroids is helpful and may be justified. Only short courses should be given for up to 4, or at the most 6, weeks.

Oestrogens and the Contraceptive Pill

Undoubtedly, the administration of oestrogenic compounds in adequate dosage to prevent ovulation improves acne in younger women. Oestrogens will help men too, but their use in males is probably never justified, as in order to obtain a clinical response a degree of feminization is an inevitable side-effect. The contraceptive pill has been occasionally used, but probably because of the progestogenic constituents the effect is unpredictable and depends on the particular preparation used. Strauss and Pochi (1964) found that a combination of norethynodrel and mestranol was often helpful after the first two or three cycles.

Other Systemic Treatments

a. Vitamin A in high dosage was fashionable at one time but this treatment appears ineffective and potentially hazardous.

b. Antiandrogenic compounds have been used recently but without dramatic success. 17-alpha-methyl-B-nortestosterone was used by Nelson and Rakoff (1970) in the treatment of hirsutism and acne and they found a good response.

c. Propanalol, tolbutamide and enzyme preparations have also been used without good effect.

Physical Methods of Treatment

Ultraviolet light (both natural and artificial) is often beneficial. The usual explanation is that ultraviolet light produces desquamation but the benefit often far outweighs any peeling action and it seems there may be another mechanism. A 6-week course of increasing twice-weekly doses is simple and often effective. The aim should be just to produce a very slight pinkness and peeling.

Strauss and Kligman (1959) thought that X-rays helped acne by suppression of the sebaceous glands. Jelliffe et al. (1969) in a controlled investigation could not demonstrate any therapeutic effect with Grenz rays or with 29-kV irradiation and only marginal benefit with 50-kV X-rays.

Treatment of Cysts

Aspiration by a wide-gauge needle is often attempted but this is usually ineffective as the contents are too viscous. Emptying the contents by a stab incision can produce considerable relief. For cysts that are not under too much tension, instillation of 0·5–1 ml triamcinolone acetonide suspension (10 mg/ml) is surprisingly effective in aiding the resolution of cysts. Cysts may also be flattened by application of a solid carbon dioxide snow stick for periods of up to 1 minute. This is painful but quite useful in flattening cysts.

Surgery

Enthusiastic surgical interference produces scars, does not aid resolution and is to be avoided.

REFERENCES

Andrews G. C. (1965) Acne vulgaris. *Med. Clin. North Am.* **49**, 737.

Baillie A. H., Thomson J. and Milne J. A. (1966) The distribution of hydroxysteroid dehydrogenases in human sebaceous glands. *Br. J. Dermatol.* **78**, 451.

Barsone G. and Reisnes R. M. (1971) Differential rates of conversion of testosterone to dihydrotestosterone in acne and in normal skin—a possible pathogenetic factor in acne. *J. Invest. Dermatol.* **56**, 316.

Beveridge G. W. and Powell E. W. (1969) Sebum changes in acne vulgaris treated with tetracycline. *Br. J. Dermatol.* **81**, 525.

Blair C. and Lewis C. A. (1970) The pigment of comedones. *Br. J. Dermatol.* **82**, 572.

Bowyer A. (1965) Fringe or pop acne. *Br. Med. J.* **2**, 1548.

Burton J. L. (1970) The physical properties of sebum in acne vulgaris. *Clin. Sci.* **39**, 757.

Calman K. C., Muir A. V., Milne J. A. and Young H. (1970) Survey of the distribution of steroid dehydrogenases in sebaceous glands of human skin. *Br. J. Dermatol* **82**, 567.

Cornelius C. E. and Ludwig G. D. (1967) Red fluorescence of comedones. Production of porphyrins by *Corynebacterium acnes*. *J. Invest. Dermatol.* **49**, 368.

Crounse R. G. (1965) The response of acne to placebos and antibiotics. *JAMA* **193**, 906.

Crow K. D. (1970) Chloracne. A critical review including a comparison of two series of cases of acne from chlornaphthalene and pitch fumes. *Trans. Rep. St John's Hosp. Dermatol. Soc.* **56**, 79.

Cunliffe W. J., Forster R. A., Greenwood N. D. et al. (1973) Tetracycline and acne vulgaris—a clinical and laboratory investigation. *Br. Med. J.* **4**, 332.

Cunliffe W. J. and Shuster S. (1969) Pathogenesis of acne. *Lancet* **1**, 685.

Damon A. (1957) Constitutional factors in acne vulgaris. *Arch. Dermatol.* **76**, 172.

Downing D. T., Strauss J. S. and Pochi P. E. (1969) Variability in the chemical composition of human surface lipids. *J. Invest. Dermatol.* **53**, 322.

Ebling F. J. (1954) Changes in the sebaceous glands and epidermis during the oestrous cycle of the albino rat. *J. Endocrinol.* **10**, 147.

Forbes H. A. W. (1946) The incidence of clinical acne in men. *Br. J. Dermatol.* **58**, 298.

Freinkel R. K. (1969) Pathogenesis of acne vulgaris. *N. Engl. J. Med.* **280**, 1161.

Freinkel R. K., Strauss J. S., Yip S. Y. and Pochi P. E. (1965) Effect of tetracycline on the composition of sebum in acne vulgaris. *N. Engl. J. Med.* **273**, 850.

Fry L. and Ramsay C. A. (1966) Tetracycline in acne vulgaris. Clinical evaluation and the effect of sebum production. *Br. J. Dermatol.* **78**, 653.

Fulton J. E., McGinley K., Leyden J. and Marples R. R. (1968) Gram-negative folliculitis in acne vulgaris. *Arch. Dermatol.* **97**, 349.

Fulton J. E., Plewig G. and Kligman A. M. (1969) Effect of chocolate on acne vulgaris. *JAMA* **210**, 2071.

Goltz R. W. and Kjartansson S. (1966) Oral tetracycline treatment on bacterial flora in acne vulgaris. *Arch. Dermatol.* **93**, 92.

Goolamali S. K., Burton J. L. and Shuster S. (1973) Sebum excretion in hypopituitarism. *Br. J. Dermatol.* **89**, 21.

Gougerot H., Carteaud A. and Grupper E. (1945) Epidémie de comédones par les brillantines, crêmes, etc. de gérer. *Bull. Soc. Fr. Dermatol. Syphiligr.* **52**, 124.

Grant J. D. and Anderson P. C. (1965) Chocolate as a cause of acne. A dissenting view. *Mo. Med.* **62**, 459.

Grant R. N. R. (1957) The relationship between acne and hair growth. *Arch. Dermatol.* **76**, 179.

Greene R., Burrell M. W. and Ivy A. C. (1939) Progesterone is androgenic. *Endocrinology* **24**, 351.

Haskin D., Lasher N. and Rothman S. (1953) Some effects of ACTH, cortisone, progesterone and testosterone on sebaceous glands in the white rat. *J. Invest. Dermatol.* **20**, 207.

Hellier F. F. (1954) Acneiform eruptions in infancy. *Br. J. Dermatol.* **66**, 25.

Herxheimer K. (1899) Über Chloracne. *Münch. Med. Wochenschr.* **46**, 278.

Izumi A. K., Marples R. R. and Kligman A. M. (1970) Bacteriology of acne comedones. *Arch. Dermatol.* **102**, 397.

Jarrett A. (1955) The effects of stilboestrol on the surface sebum and upon acne vulgaris. *Br. J. Dermatol.* **67**, 165.

Jelliffe A. M., Soutter C., and Meara R. H. (1969) An investigation into the treatment of acne vulgaris with Grenz X-rays. *Br. J. Dermatol.* **81**, 617.

Jones J. W. and Alden H. S. (1936) An acneiform dermatergosis. *Arch. Dermatol.* **33**, 1022.

Katsuki et al. (1969) Reports of the study for 'Yusho' (chlorbiphenyl poisoning), June 1969. Study group for Yusho, Faculty of Medicine, Kyushu University, Fukuoka, Japan. *Acta Med. (Fukuoka)*.

Kellum R. E. (1967) Human sebaceous gland lipids. *Arch. Dermatol.* **95**, 218.

Kellum R. E. (1968) Acne vulgaris. Studies in pathogenesis. Relative irritancy of free fatty acids from C_2 to C_{16}. *Arch. Dermatol.* **97**, 722.

Kellum R. E. and Strangfeld K. (1970) Acne vulgaris. Studies in pathogenesis. Fatty acids of *Corynebacterium acnes*. *Arch. Dermatol.* **101**, 337.

Kellum R. E. and Strangfeld K. (1972) Acne vulgaris. Studies in pathogenesis. Fatty acids of human surface triglycerides from patients with and without acne. *J. Invest. Dermatol.* **58**, 315.

Kellum R. E., Strangfeld K. and Ray L. F. (1970) Acne vulgaris. Studies in pathogenesis. Triglyceride hydrolysis by *C. acnes in vitro*. *Arch. Dermatol.* **101**, 41.

Kenyon F. E. (1966) Psychosomatic aspects of acne. *Br. J. Dermatol.* **78**, 344.

Kligman A. M., Fulton J. E. and Plewig G. (1969) Topical vitamin A acid in acne vulgaris. *Arch. Dermatol.* **99**, 469.

Kligman A. M. and Mills O. (1972) Acne cosmetica. *Arch. Dermatol.* **106**, 843.

Kligman A. M., Wheatley V. R. and Mills O. H. (1970) Comedogenicity of human sebum. *Arch. Dermatol.* **102**, 267.

Krakow R., Downing D. T., Strauss J. S. and Pochi P. E. (1973) Identification of a fatty acid in human skin surface lipids apparently associated with acne vulgaris. *J. Invest. Dermatol.* **61**, 286.

Lane P. and Williamson D. M. (1969) Treatment of acne vulgaris with tetracycline hydrochloride: a double-blind trial with 51 patients. *Br. Med. J.* **2**, 76.

Lever W. F and Lever G. S. (1975) *Histopathology of the Skin*, 5th ed. Philadelphia, Lippincott.

Lipkin G., Wheatley V. R., Tae Ha Woo and March C. (1968) Studies of the lipids of dog skin. IV. The *in vivo* incorporation of blood lipids into the lipids of isolated perfused dog skin. *J. Invest. Dermatol.* **50**, 456.

Lucas C. J. (1961) Personality of students with acne vulgaris. *Br. Med. J.* **11**, 354.

Lynch F. W. (1940) Acne vulgaris: review of histological changes observed in early lesions. *Arch. Dermatol.* **42**, 593.

MacDonald I. (1968) Effects of a skimmed milk and chocolate diet on serum and skin lipids. *J. Sci. Food Agric.* **19**, 270.

Maibach H. (1967) Pustules due to *Corynebacterium acnes*. *Arch. Dermatol.* **96**, 453.

Marks R. and Davies M. J. (1969) The distribution in the skin of systemically administered tetracycline. *Br. J. Dermatol.* **81**, 448.

Marples R. R., Downing D. T. and Kligman A. M. (1972) Influence of *Pityrosporon* species in the generation of free fatty acids in human surface lipids. *J. Invest. Dermatol.* **58**, 155.

Marples R. R., Fulton J. E., Leyden J. and McGinley K. J. (1969) Effect of antibiotics on the nasal flora in acne patients. *Arch. Dermatol.* **99**, 647.

Marples R. R. and Izumi A. K. (1970) Bacteriology of pustular acne. *J. Invest. Dermatol.* **54**, 252.

Marples R. R. and Kligman A. M. (1971) Ecological effects of oral antibiotics on the microflora of human skin. *Arch. Dermatol.* **103**, 148.

Mills O. and Kligman A. M. (1972) Is sulphur harmful? *Br. J. Dermatol.* **86**, 620.

Munro-Ashman D. (1963) Acne vulgaris in a public school. *Trans. Rep. St John's Hosp. Dermatol. Soc.* **49**, 144.

Nelson R. M. and Rakoff A. E. (1970) Hirsutism and acne treated by an androgen antagonist. *Obstet. Gynecol.* **36**, 748.

Newman B. A. and Feldman F. F. (1954) Adult premenstrual acne. An entity suggesting corpus luteum dysfunction. *Arch. Dermatol.* **69**, 356.

Nicolaides N. and Wells G. C. (1957) On the biogenesis of the free fatty acids in human skin surface fat. *J. Invest. Dermatol.* **29**, 423.

Olansky S. (1967) Re-evaluation of sulphacetamide as a topical agent in the treatment of pustular acne. *Cutis* **3**, 613.

Pace W. E. (1965) A benzoyl peroxide-sulphur cream for acne vulgaris. *Can. Med. Assoc. J.* **93**, 252.

Pinkus H. and Mehregan A. H. (1969) *A Guide to Dermatohistopathology.* New York, Appleton-Century-Crofts.

Plewig G. (1974) Acne vulgaris—proliferative cells in sebaceous glands. *Br. J. Dermatol.* **90**, 623.

Plewig G., Fulton J. E. and Kligman A. M. (1970) Pomade acne. *Arch. Dermatol.* **101**, 580.

Plewig G., Petrozzi J. W. and Berendes U. (1970) Double-blind study of doxycycline in acne vulgaris. *Arch. Dermatol.* **101**, 435.

Pochi P. E., Downing D. T. and Strauss J. S. (1970) Sebaceous gland response in man to prolonged total calorie deprivation. *J. Invest. Dermatol.* **55**, 303.

Pochi P. E. and Strauss J. S. (1964) Sebum production, casual sebum levels, titratable acidity of sebum and urinary fractional 17 keto-steroid excretion in males with acne. *J. Invest. Dermatol.* **43**, 383.

Pochi P. E. and Strauss J. S. (1967) Effect of prednisone on sebaceous gland secretion. *J. Invest. Dermatol.* **49**, 456.

Pochi P. E., Strauss J. S., Rao G. S., Sanda J. R., Forchielle E. and Dorfman R. I. (1965) Plasma testosterone and oestrogen levels, urine testosterone excretion and sebum production in males with acne vulgaris. *J. Clin. Endocrinol.* **25**, 1660.

Powell E. W. (1970) The effects of 2-naphthol peeling paste on sebaceous glands remote from its site of application. *Br. J. Dermatol.* **82**, 371.

Powell E. W. and Beveridge G. W. (1970) Sebum excretion and sebum composition in adolescent men with and without acne vulgaris. *Br. J. Dermatol.* **82**, 243.

Power K. (1970) Complications from combined oral tetracycline and oral corticoid therapy in acne vulgaris. *Med. J. Aust.* **1**, 1059.

Puhvel S. M., Barfatani M., Warnick M. and Sternberg T. H. (1964) Study of antibody levels to *Corynebacterium acnes. Arch. Dermatol.* **90**, 421.

Puhvel S. M. and Reisner R. M. (1972) The production of hyaluronidase by *C. acnes. J. Invest. Dermatol.* **58**, 66.

Puhvel S. M., Warnick M. A. and Sternberg T. H. (1965) Levels of antibody to *Staphylococcus epidermidis* in patients with acne vulgaris. *Arch. Dermatol.* **92**, 88.

Ratzer M. A. (1964) The influence of marriage, pregnancy and childbirth on acne vulgaris. *Br. J. Dermatol.* **76**, 165.

Robinson R. C. V. (1964) Long term therapy of acne with sulphadimethoxine: toxicity studies. *South. Med. J.* **57**, 655.

Rook A. J., Wilkinson D. S. and Ebling F. J. G. (1972) *Textbook of Dermatology,* 2nd ed., vol. 2. Oxford, Blackwell Scientific, pp. 1545–1558.

Rosenberg E. W. (1969) Bacteriology of acne. *Annu. Rev. Med.* **20**, 201.

Sabouraud R. (1897) *Ann. Inst. Pasteur* **11**, 134.

Savin R. C. and Turner M. C. (1966) Antibiotics and the placebo reaction in acne. *JAMA* **196**, 365.

Schwartz L., Tulipan L. and Peck S. M. (1947) *Occupational Diseases of the Skin,* 2nd ed. Philadelphia, Lea & Febiger.

Shalita A. R. and Wheatley V. (1970) Inhibition of pancreatic lipase by tetracyclines. *J. Invest. Dermatol.* **54**, 413.

Shehadeh N. H. and Kligman A. M. (1963) The bacteriology of acne. *Arch. Dermatol.* **88**, 829.

Shelley W. B. and Kligman A. M. (1957) The experimental production of acne by penta and hexachloronaphthalenes. *Arch. Dermatol.* **75**, 689.

Smith M. A. and Waterworth P. M. (1961) The bacteriology of acne vulgaris in relation to its treatment with antibiotics. *Br. J. Dermatol.* **73**, 152.

Smith M. A., Waterworth P. M. and Curwen M. P. (1962) A controlled trial of oral antibiotics in the treatment of acne vulgaris. *Br. J. Dermatol.* **74**, 86.

Stafford I., Cunliffe W. J., Tubman J. and Hall R. (1969) Serum growth hormone in patients with acne vulgaris. *Br. J. Dermatol.* **81**, 909.

Strauss J. S. and Kligman A. M. (1959) Effect of X-rays on sebaceous glands of the human face. Radiation therapy of acne. *J. Invest. Dermatol.* **33**, 348.

Strauss J. S. and Kligman A. M. (1956) Acne: observations on dermabrasion and the anatomy of the acne pit. *Arch. Dermatol.* **74**, 397.

Strauss J. S. and Kligman A. M. (1960) The pathologic dynamics of acne vulgaris. *Arch. Dermatol.* **82**, 779.

Strauss J. S. and Kligman A. M. (1961) The effect of progesterone and progesterone-like compounds on the human sebaceous gland. *J. Invest. Dermatol.* **36**, 309.

Strauss J. S., Kligman A. M. and Pochi P. E. (1962) The effect of androgens and oestrogens on human sebaceous glands. *J. Invest. Dermatol.* **36**, 293.

Strauss J. S. and Pochi P. E. (1964) Effect of cyclic progestin oestrogen therapy on sebum and acne in women. *JAMA* **190**, 815.

Strauss J. S. and Pochi P. E. (1965) Intracutaneous injection of sebum and comedones. *Arch. Dermatol.* **92**, 443.

Tzanck A., Slide E. and Dobkevitch S. (1945) Nombreux cas d'éruption acnéiforme provoqués par une brillantine de fabrication récente. *Bull. Soc. Fr. Dermatol. Syphiligr.* **52**, 131.

Unna P. G. (1896) *The Histopathology of the Diseases of the Skin.* Edinburgh, Clay pp. 352–366.

Van Scott E. S. and McCardle R. C. (1956) Keratinisation of the duct of the sebaceous gland and growth cycle of the hair follicle in the histogenesis of acne in human skin. *J. Invest. Dermatol.* **27**, 405.

Vasarinsh P. (1969) Keratinisation of pilar structures in acne vulgaris and normal skin. *Br. J. Dermatol.* **81**, 517.

Watson J. B. (1959) Monoporous and polyporous acne. *Arch. Dermatol.* **80**, 167.

Weary P. E., Russell C. M., Butter H. K. and Hsu Y. T. (1969) Acneiform eruption resulting from antibiotic administration. *Arch. Dermatol.* **100**, 179.

Chapter 5

Dermatitis of the Face

In this chapter the clinical patterns of dermatitis affecting the face will be discussed. The term 'eczema' and 'dermatitis' will be regarded as synonymous here.

It should be remembered that eczematous change represents a reaction pattern of the epidermis to a number of different sorts of injury. The challenge lies in finding the precipitating cause and in eventually removing it.

ATOPIC DERMATITIS

Atopy in one form or another affects up to 20 per cent of the Caucasian population (Carr et al., 1964). Atopic dermatitis affects all racial groups; it seems to be common in American Negroes, and Kenney (1965) found that it occurred in 11·7 per cent of 3800 Negro patients.

Definition

An inherited form of dermatitis characterized by pruritus, and the tendency to lichenification (often with a characteristic flexural predilection) which may be associated with asthma and/or hay fever and in which the presence of reaginic antibodies can be identified in the serum.

Clinical Picture on the Face

The Atopic Facies. The atopic facies is more easily recognized than described. A good example is seen in *Fig.* 34. In part it is the lichenification around the eyes and the comparative pallor of the malar regions that makes the face distinctive. In addition there appears to be an anomalous fold around the eye similar to an epicanthic fold.

In atopic dermatitis, the face and neck are not infrequently affected and can be a very troublesome part of the overall picture. In children particularly, there may be exuding crusted patches involving the cheeks, ears and scalp (*Fig.* 35). It is common for these crusted patches to be misdiagnosed as impetigo. It should be remembered that oozing and crusting are an integral part of eczema and the equation 'yellow crusts = antibiotics' is basically incorrect. In young adults a different picture may be seen, with lichenification particularly around the eyes and around the lower jaw and with persistent pinkness of the face as well. On the neck there is sometimes a pronounced brown reticulated pigmentation and follicular prominence (*Plate* 5B). This is similar to the condition described as 'erythromelanosis follicularis faciei et colli' by Mishima and Rudner (1966). It does not seem to be poikilodermatous and its causation is unknown. It may be merely lichenification with exaggeration of the normal skin markings.

SEBORRHOEIC DERMATITIS

This variety of eczema is extremely common. It seems to affect Caucasians and especially European Caucasians more than other racial groups. Most ages are affected, though it is not often seen in prepubertal children.

Definition
A type of constitutional eczema in which the large body flexures and intertriginous zones are particularly involved.

The inadequacy of this definition is obvious. It is a term employed for a number of clinical situations and in all probability does not represent a single pathogenetic process.

Clinical Picture on the Face
A common story is that of a patient with mild dandruff for some months who then develops scaliness of the eyebrows, a mild persistent marginal blepharitis and some pinkness and scaliness of the nasolabial grooves. Other areas that might become involved include the retro-auricular areas, the external ear itself and the neck. The scalp margin might become affected. The disorder is subject to spontaneous remissions and relapses, so that caution should be employed before accepting the effectiveness of any one particular treatment or the validity of the patient's explanation for the cause of a relapse. It is common for patients with this complaint to suggest that the cause of their rash is 'emotional stress'. There is no firm evidence to support this contention.

It is sometimes very difficult to distinguish this type of chronic persistent eczema from psoriasis. The clinical appearances may be very similar. This seems especially true for middle-aged men and the facetious term 'seborrhiasis' has been coined to describe this situation. Usually there is also patchy pink scaliness on the scalp and face with dull red indolently scaling plaques on the upper trunk.

There are other less well-defined clinical situations where the term 'seborrhoeic dermatitis' is used by the clinician. An acute exudative type of eczema, affecting the ears particularly and sometimes called 'infectious eczematoid dermatitis', is one such condition. When discoid patches also occur on the face and become crusted, they are often mistaken for impetigo (*Fig.* 36). The term *seborrhoeic folliculitis* is sometimes used as an excuse for a more thoughtful diagnosis in patients with a sparse indolent papular rash on the beard area and over the back. In many cases where this diagnosis has been made, it would be better to regard the disorder as a type of acne or pyococcal folliculitis.

Because the concept of seborrhoeic dermatitis is so indistinct it is as well to exclude other conditions that may appear similar, before making the diagnosis. The following should be especially considered in *differential diagnosis*.

a. Psoriasis.
b. Superficial pemphigus.
c. Impetigo.
d. Hailey–Hailey pemphigus.
e. Darier's disease.
f. Acne.
g. Rosacea.
h. Perioral dermatitis.

CONTACT DERMATITIS

Allergic Contact Dermatitis of the Face
Acute allergic contact dermatitis may present an extremely dramatic picture (*Plate* 6A). The whole face may be red and puffy and oozing in places. The eyelids, in particular, take the brunt of the inflammatory process, and may swell so much that it becomes impossible to open the eyes. Less severe reactions are, however, more commonly seen and are characterized by excoriated or lichenified pink and scaly patches affecting areas such as the eyelids, the periorbital regions or the forehead. The subject of contact dermatitis of the face has been extensively reviewed and discussed by Sidi (1962).

Reactions due to Cosmetics
It is difficult to obtain any accurate figures for the overall incidence of allergic contact dermatitis due to cosmetics in the community. It is probable that many minor reactions remain unreported and the sufferer merely ceases using the particular product that she (or he) has identified as being responsible. In addition, many reactions are treated successfully by the general practitioner and never come to the notice of dermatologists. Hjorth (1959) found that 2 per cent of patients with

8

eczematous reactions had an allergic contact dermatitis to a cosmetic product confirmed by patch testing.

However, it is also true that many patients with persistent eczema of the face—particularly the eyelids—unjustly blame some perfectly innocuous cosmetic product. Kaalund-Jorgenson (1951) found that less than 25 per cent of a group of patients with dermatitis of the eyelids had a reaction due to a beauty product. When a hypersensitivity reaction to a cosmetic is suspected, Fisher (1967) suggests that a 'cosmetic elimination test' is employed to identify the offending agent. In this procedure all cosmetics are avoided and reintroduced one at a time. Patch testing may also be employed but a 'use test' may well be more sensitive in determining the cause. This is due to the very sensitive nature of the skin of the face compared to that of the usual patch test sites on the back. Furthermore, there may be special qualities of the cosmetic formulation used that have caused a reaction (such as coincidental presence of a primary irritant enhancing a weak sensitizer); these qualities may not be present in the individual constituents used in patch testing.

Nail Varnish. It may be surprising that preparations applied to the finger-nails should be responsible for eczematous reactions on the face and neck and only rarely affect the paronychial tissues. The eyelids and the sides of the neck are primarily involved and presumably their localization is due to the frequent touching of these sites and to the sensitivity of the region. If undiagnosed, other areas may later become affected. The ingredients responsible are usually sulphonamide-formaldehyde resins. Occasionally one of the fluorescent dyes used as a colouring agent is responsible, e.g. eosin or fluorescein. Formaldehyde in nail hardeners and acrylic monomer in artificial nails are also occasionally the cause of an allergic contact dermatitis of this type.

Lipstick. Hypersensitivity to constituents of lipstick may cause a cheilitis. This has become very uncommon since the removal of the sensitizer eosin from most lipsticks. The dyes now used include the halogen derivatives of fluorescein such as tetrabromofluorescein and colour lakes from the precipitation of soluble dyes with aluminium or calcium salts. These rarely sensitize. Other ingredients such as cocoa, butter and perfumes may occasionally act as sensitizers in lipsticks.

Eye Make-ups. The sensitizers responsible in mascara and other preparations include various pigments, dyes, perfumes and resins as well as preservatives.

Hair Preparations. Phenolic compounds such as chlorothymol, resorcinol and betanaphthol are sometimes found in hair tonics and are potential sensitizers. Eugenol, a constituent of oil of bay (found in the vehicle bay-rum), is quite a strong sensitizer. Other oils and perfumes may be the cause of an allergic contact dermatitis on rare occasions. Dermatitis caused by these products affects the scalp, forehead, the ears and the back of the neck.

One of the commonest types of allergic contact dermatitis from cosmetic products is that due to *paraphenylenediamine* (PPD). This dye requires oxidation to become coloured and the oxidizer (which is often hydrogen peroxide) is supplied in a separate container. It can produce a very florid dermatitis affecting the scalp and the whole face. Often the forehead and eyelids are affected and there may be streaky dermatitis running down the face as well. A routine open patch test is recommended by the manufacturers to be applied to a small area for 24 hours before use of the dye to detect those with hypersensitivity. PPD cross-reacts with a number of compounds including sulphonamides and some local anaesthetics and anyone who has developed a hair dermatitis should be acquainted with this possibility. Other less frequently used dyes are sometimes contact sensitizers, including paratoluenediamine and the azo dyes.

Miscellaneous Products. Bleaching creams containing monobenzyl ether of hydroquinone and hydroquinone may produce a very severe dermatitic rash with eventual profound depigmentation and a severe cosmetic defect as a consequence. Ammoniated mercury which is present in some depigmenting creams is also sometimes responsible for allergic contact dermatitis. *Lanolin* is present in many creams and lotions as a base and is a not uncommon cause of allergic contact dermatitis (*see below*). *Perfumes* are also an occasional cause of sensitization; there are literally thousands of these in commercial use and sorting out which is responsible may be an impossible task. *Balsam of Peru* is another frequently used aromatic compound that frequently causes allergic contact dermatitis. The balsams have recently been found to be the commonest of all allergens tested in patients with eczema in a co-operative European survey (Fregert et al., 1969). *Dental preparations* may produce a cheilitis and a perioral eczema. The sensitizing compounds include essential oils and antiseptics such as dichlorophene, 8-hydroxyquinoline and nitrofurazone. However, this is an extremely uncommon occurrence.

Reactions due to Medicaments
These reactions are becoming increasingly common; 15 per cent of patients with allergic contact dermatitis were found by Fregert et al. (1969) to have contracted the condition through use of an applied medicament. It should be remembered that ophthalmic preparations and also topical treatments for the ears are often the cause of a persistent dermatitis, due to their content of sensitizing compounds. *Neomycin* has been a frequent cause of contact dermatitis but has been amongst the

most difficult of contact hypersensitivities to recognize. The difficulties arose because of the frequent use of neomycin in combination with corticosteroids and the consequent masking of the acute eczematous response (Epstein, 1965). In addition, neomycin appears to evoke an undramatic eczematous picture and patch tests with this antibiotic have to be performed with especial care. Twenty per cent preparations should be used, and even then delayed positives may be seen which can easily be missed. Neomycin sensitivity is a frequent cause of persistent periocular eczema and otitis externa from the use of eye and ear preparations containing this antibiotic. *Lanolin* (*see also above*, under Reactions due to Cosmetics) is a frequent cause of dermatitis medicamentosa. It is not uncommon for patients to be sensitive to both lanolin and neomycin. Cronin (1966) reviews the subject of lanolin sensitivity comprehensively, and suggests either the applications of 30 per cent wood alcohols in yellow soft paraffin or unguentum aquosum BP with plastic film occlusion as patch test procedures. Lanolin is a most complex material and there may be several sensitizing compounds in it. Women seem to be more prone to lanolin sensitivity and this may be because of their more frequent contact with lanolin in cosmetics. As with neomycin, recognition of lanolin sensitivity is often needlessly delayed because it is not considered. Lanolin is a constituent of most ointments and many creams and if applied as a corticosteroid preparation the local acute eczematous response resulting may well be suppressed. *Iodochlorhydroxy quinoline* (Vioform)—it used to be thought that this antimicrobial compound was not a sensitizer; this proved to be a false hope. It accounts for a substantial number of patients with dermatitis medicamentosa and is included in the 'standard battery' of patch test materials in the contact clinic at St John's Hospital for Diseases of the Skin. *Parabens* (esters of parahydroxybenzoic acid) are used as preservatives in many creams because of their antimicrobial properties. They are sensitizers, but they cause less trouble here than in Scandinavia where they were used in higher concentrations as topical fungistatic agents.

There is a variety of other occasionally sensitizing materials used in topical preparations. *Diphenhydramine cream* is a popular 'anti-allergic' nostrum which is sometimes the cause of contact dermatitis. Despite its widespread use there is neither theoretical nor clinical evidence of the effectiveness of this preparation. *Chloroxylenols* (*Dettol*) are popular household disinfectants also capable of sensitization. *Mercurial compounds* and the '-*caine*' local anaesthetics are also sensitizers (especially the latter group) but luckily are being decreasingly used.

Sidi (1962) in his discussion on eczema of the face due to medications also mentions airborne materials, especially penicillin and streptomycin. These sometimes cause an extraordinarily high degree of sensitivity, especially in nurses who 'draw up' these materials for injection. It may become impossible for them to walk into a ward in which these treatments are being used.

Miscellaneous Sensitizers

Primula. Sensitivity to this family of flowers produces a violent eczematous response in some patients. A very high degree of sensitivity may be found with episodes of facial swelling and dermatitis from minimal or indirect contact with the plant. The subject has been well reviewed by Hjorth (1966). The sensitizing capacity of the primula plant depends on the season, as does its content of the actual sensitizing compound 'primulin'. The leaves contain more of this compound than do the flower. The particular species most often responsible for this type of contact dermatitis is *Primula obconica. Chrysanthemums* and *geraniums* are other plants that are occasionally the cause of a facial dermatitis. There are others that sensitize the rare unlucky individual and they may be very difficult to pinpoint. This is especially true if the allergen is airborne such as it is with a dermatitis seen in West Canadian woodsmen. The cause was eventually tracked down to lichen growing on the trees of the locality and the sensitizing compound has been found to be usnic acid (Mitchell, 1965).

Strike anywhere matches contain phosphorus sesquisulphide and Ive (1967) described seven patients with an eczematous rash from this compound. These matches can cause recurrent facial eczema from the combustion products of the struck match or eczema of the thigh under the pocket in which the matches are usually carried. They can also be the cause of a hand eczema.

Industrial airborne allergens are particularly important as a cause of facial dermatitis. *Wood dusts*—for example, rosewood or mahogany— may be responsible. *Resins*—such as epoxy resin—and various *rubber additives* and *accelerators* should be mentioned here (*Fig. 37*).

Spectacle frames are sometimes the cause of a persistent eczema where they are in direct contact with the skin. Tricresyl phosphate and triphenyl phosphate are plasticizers that have been incriminated in some patients as the responsible sensitizers (Smith and Calnan, 1966). It should be remembered that nickel in metal frames may be the allergen at fault.

Finally, in discussing allergic contact dermatitis of the face it must be said that there are patients who develop acute eczematous rashes on the face in a distribution suggestive of an airborne sensitizer but for which no particular allergen is identified. An exacting history and a painstaking search are worthwhile as only in this way is the cause likely to be found. (Photocontact dermatitis will be dealt with in Chapter 7.)

Contact Dermatitis of the Face due to Primary Irritants

Apart from inadvertent exposure to either acids or alkalis, primary irritant dermatitis of the face is usually due to some sort of therapeutic or cosmetic application. *Sulphur* preparations may prove irritating and some individuals appear prone to this side-effect (*Fig.* 38). *Benzoyl peroxide* can also be responsible for an irritant dermatitis. *Calcium* (or *ammonium*) *thioglycollate* and *calcium hydroxide* in depilatory preparations if left on the face for longer than the recommended time may cause a dermatitis. Depilatory preparations are usually alkaline with a pH of 11–12·5 and this contributes to the potential irritancy. Permanent waving solutions also contain thioglycollates and may be the cause of an irritant dermatitis. Other materials that can cause a primary irritant dermatitis include hexachlorophene solutions and various quaternary ammonium compounds (including Cetavlon). The former has been described as causing a scrotal dermatitis (Baker et al., 1969) and some patients with acne are made quite sore from its use.

PITYRIASIS SIMPLEX (Pityriasis alba)

This condition is an extremely common facial rash seen in young children and also occasionally in young adults. Characteristically there are pale pink or even whitish discoid areas on the lower face (*Fig.* 39). All racial groups seem to be affected but it is particularly noticeable in Negro subjects as the affected areas often appear slightly depigmented. The cause is unknown and, contrary to earlier thought, no particular micro-organism has been found responsible. The condition is extraordinarily persistent and resists most of the usual treatment for eczema. Recently, two families have been observed at St John's Hospital in whom several members were affected.

LIP-LICKING CHEILITIS

Children who obsessionally run their tongue around their lips develop a curious patterned dermatitis which vanishes when they stop this habit (*Fig.* 40).

PITYRIASIS ROSEA

This occurs on the face more commonly than is sometimes thought. Cohen (1967) found that pityriasiform macules occurred on the forehead of 15 per cent of those affected (*Fig.* 41). Lesions may also occur in the frontal part of the scalp.

DERMATITIS ARTEFACTA

Self-inflicted injury to the skin is frequently seen on the face because of its accessibility and its importance for the individual as a means of communication. Such lesions may be eczematous in type from the application of primary irritants (*Plate* 6B). Alkalis and acids of various types are sometimes the culprits but almost any irritant material may be used including pumice and fibreglass.

Erosions and ulcerated lesions are also typical of lesions of dermatitis artefacta but the types of lesions seen vary enormously. Dermatitis artefacta can be difficult to recognize. The bizarre shapes of the lesion are an important pointer to the diagnosis. Furthermore, the lesions tend to be asymmetrical and in unusual anatomical distributions. There is also often a striking lack of surrounding inflammation near the eroded lesions. The excoriated papular lesions on the forehead and cheeks seen in patients with acne are not the same thing and have a different significance and a better prognosis.

Patients with dermatitis artefacta are usually of an hysterical personality type and their social background should be carefully assessed. Unfortunately, these patients rarely seem to benefit from psychiatric attention.

Injection of alcohol into the Gasserian ganglion for the relief of trigeminal neuralgia sometimes leaves the subject with persistent and distressing paraesthesiae with accompanying hypo-aesthesia. This can occasionally lead to a remarkable artefactual type of lesion which is refractory to all treatments (*see* Chapter 10).

DIFFERENTIAL DIAGNOSIS OF FACIAL ECZEMA

1. *Psoriasis.* The lesions of psoriasis are sometimes seen on the face, particularly at the sides of the nose, in the eyebrows and on the hair line. The lesions are well defined and have a thicker scale than eczematous lesions.

2. *Ringworm* (*see below* in Chapter 8). This should always be considered. Direct microscopical examination for fungus is relatively easy and there is little excuse for not doing it in patients with slightly atypical 'eczema' of limited extent. Careful search will usually reveal an 'edge' in ringworm.

3. *Pityriasis versicolor.* This may occur as small pale scaly patches on the lower face and neck. Diagnosis is easily made by examining the scale microscopically.

4. *Rosacea.* There may be genuine difficulty in distinguishing mild rosacea from facial seborrhoeic dermatitis in some patients. This is especially true if, in a patient with rosacea, there are only a few

scattered papules and only a mild erythema and some dandruff in addition.

5. *Perioral dermatitis.* If this rash is limited to the nasolabial folds confusion with seborrhoeic dermatitis is possible. The presence of small papules, the lack of response to topical corticosteroids and the absence of any signs of seborrhoeic dermatitis elsewhere distinguishes perioral dermatitis.

6. *Patches of discoid lupus erythematosus.* These are fixed, well marginated and show atrophy but in the early stages may easily be confused with patches of eczema.

7. *Impetigo.* This disorder occurs in well-defined patches and is of limited extent. There is a characteristic moist golden crust and in the early stages blisters may be seen. The difficulty in distinguishing this disorder from exudative eczema has already been mentioned.

8. *Superficial pemphigus*, and *Darier's disease*, should be considered in crusted scaling conditions.

TREATMENT OF FACIAL ECZEMA

Avoidance of any proven causative sensitizers or primary irritants is of prime importance. In general powerful corticosteroids should only be used when weaker measures have failed. Simple bland creams may suffice; seborrhoeic dermatitis may respond to sulphur and salicylic acid ointment (BNF). Hydrocortisone preparations or diluted proprietary preparations of powerful corticosteroids (e.g. 1 in 4) are satisfactory for the vast majority of patients with eczema. If powerful corticosteroids are used then the possibility of severe atrophy occurring as a side-effect should be borne in mind. It is helpful to recommend the use of emulsifying ointment BNF instead of soap which may irritate eczematous areas.

REFERENCES

Baker H., Ive F. A. and Lloyd M. J. (1969) Primary irritant dermatitis of the scrotum due to hexachlorophene. *Arch. Dermatol.* **99**, 693.

Carr R. D., Berke M. and Becker S. W. (1964) Incidence of atopy in the general population. *Arch. Dermatol.* **89**, 27.

Cohen E. L. (1967) Pityriasis rosea. *Br. J. Dermatol.* **79**, 533.

Cronin E. (1966) Lanolin dermatitis. *Br. J. Dermatol.* **78**, 167.

Epstein E. (1965) Detection of neomycin sensitivity. A comparison of testing techniques. *Arch. Dermatol.* **91**, 50.

Fisher A. A. (1967) *Contact Dermatitis.* Philadelphia, Lea & Febiger.

Fregert S., Hjorth N., Magnusson B. et al. (1969) Epidemiology of contact dermatitis. *Trans. St John's Hosp. Dermatol. Soc.* **55**, 17.

Hjorth N. (1959) Cosmetic allergy. *J. Soc. Cosmetic Chemists* **10**, 96.

Hjorth N. (1966) Primula dermatitis. Sources of errors in patch testing and patch test sensitisation. *Trans. St John's Hosp. Dermatol. Soc.* **52**, 207.

Ive F. A. (1967) Studies in contact dermatitis. XXI: Matches. *Trans. St John's Hosp. Dermatol. Soc.* **53**, 135.

Kaalund-Jorgenson O. (1951) Dermatitis of eyelids. *Acta Derm. Venereol. (Stockh.)* **31**, 82.

Kenney J. A. (1965) Management of dermatoses peculiar to negroes. *Arch. Dermatol.* **91**, 126.

Mishima Y. and Rudner E. (1966) Erythromelanosis follicularis faciei et colli. *Dermatologica* **132**, 269.

Mitchell J. C. (1965) Allergy to lichens. Allergic contact dermatitis from usnic acid produced by lichenized fungi. *Arch. Dermatol.* **92**, 142.

Sidi E. (1962) *Les Dermites Allergiques du Visage de Cause Externe.* Paris, L'Expansion Scientifique Française.

Smith E. L. and Calnan C. D. (1966) Studies in contact dermatitis. XVII: Spectacle frames. *Trans. St John's Hosp. Dermatol. Soc.* **52**, 10.

Chapter 6

Lupus Erythematosus and Dermatomyositis

These diseases belong to the group of disorders known as the 'connective tissue' or more recently the 'auto-immune' diseases—neither term is completely accurate and the term 'connective tissue diseases' will be used here.

LUPUS ERYTHEMATOSUS

The term 'lupus' was originally given to any persistent destructive disorder of the face. Lupus erythematosus was distinguished from lupus vulgaris at the middle of the nineteenth century by Cazenove, Hebra and Kaposi. It was at first believed to be a manifestation of tuberculosis, but later it was realized that it affected many organs and often involved blood vessels. Klemperer first introduced the term 'collagen disease' in the early 1940's (Klemperer et al., 1941).

DISCOID LUPUS ERYTHEMATOSUS

Definition

A chronic focal inflammatory disease of the skin characterized clinically by the presence of scaling, red patches that become scarred and atrophic, and in which globulin can be demonstrated (by immunofluorescence) bound to the basement membrane.

It is more common in women than in men but the quoted incidence varies from 3 : 1 to 3 : 2 (Epstein and Tuffanelli, 1966). It is most common in the 20–40-year age group but its onset has been described in patients of all ages from infancy to old age. It is not a common disease, but it is by no means rare. It accounted for about one-quarter of 1 per cent of all new patients seen at St John's Hospital for Diseases of the Skin between 1965 and 1971, while Gold (1960) found it had accounted for 0·4–0·7 per cent of new patients at the same hospital (1952–8). Lodin and Thyresson (1955) found that 1 per cent of all skin patients at the Karolinska Institute from 1948 to 1954 had some form of lupus erythematosus.

All racial groups are affected, but the relative incidence in the different groups is not known. Some have suggested that it is more common in fair Nordic types, but it seems to be common in Negroes as well. There is an increased incidence of this disease in the families of affected individuals as with all members of this group of diseases. The basis for this increased incidence is unknown. It certainly does not seem to obey any of the simple rules of inheritance.

Clinical Picture

The most commonly involved site is the face, although anywhere on the skin and even the mucosae may be involved. Gold (1960) found that the nose and cheeks were the areas most frequently affected. There is a striking predilection for the sun exposed sites. This is made dramatically obvious in some women when the ear lobe and lower part of the ear are involved, but the upper part of the ear is spared, being screened from the sun by hair. The lesions are well defined, red scaly patches (*Plate* 7A). The scale is attached at hair follicle pores and is fancifully described as 'tin-tack scaling'. There may be much atrophy and scarring especially in lesions present for a considerable length of time. Telangiectasia may be a prominent feature where there is atrophy (*Fig.* 42). Sometimes individual lesions join to form plaques with a polycyclic border. The lesions tend to spread with an active edge leaving 'healing' and scarring behind. The scarring can produce unpleasant deformities especially where the process has been extensive and persistent over the nose or cheeks. In addition, there may be irregularly mottled hyper- and hypopigmentation in and at the border of the lesions. The scalp is frequently affected and this is one cause of scarring alopecia. When the active disease has subsided the area of atrophy and hair loss produced may be difficult to distinguish from the results of lichen planus or any severe inflammatory process affecting the scalp.

The disease is remittent in character, and periods of activity and of comparative quiescence are seen. The remittent nature may be extremely noticeable in some patients, but hardly noticeable in others.

VARIANTS

Lupus Erythematosus Profundus

This type of localized lupus erythematosus (LE) is eponymously termed 'Kaposi-Irgung disease'. Fountain (1968) described 6 cases and reviewed the literature giving an excellent account of this disorder. The lesions are deep nodules or sometimes plaques and may occasionally underly ordinary patches of discoid LE. When they heal, these patches may leave considerable atrophy. The upper arms, face and scalp are most commonly involved. Although uncommon, patients with this type of lesion are more often seen than was once thought.

Hypertrophic Discoid LE

In this rare variation the lesion is a raised plaque with a rolled edge.

Disseminated Discoid Lupus Erythematosus

It is justifiable to describe this disorder as a separate type of discoid LE because the clinical pattern and behaviour are sufficiently distinctive. Typically the patient is a young or middle-aged woman with a large number of discoid lesions affecting the arms, face and sometimes the upper trunk. The light-exposed areas are particularly prone to develop large numbers of lesions. Characteristically the lesions are persistent, but not as destructive as in chronic discoid LE and some may fade without leaving a trace. Patients with disseminated discoid LE may have many of the laboratory findings of 'systemic involvement' including a neutropenia, a raised ESR, a raised level of gamma-globulin, a normochromic anaemia and a positive Coombs' test (*see below*). However, despite the laboratory findings they do not seem to develop systemic disease any more frequently than do patients with ordinary discoid LE.

COMPLICATIONS

1. Severe disfigurement from atrophy, scarring, irregular hyper- and hypopigmentation and loss of hair from the affected area.

2. The development of squamous cell carcinoma in the scar. This now seems less common than it appears to have been, and one explanation has been that this complication was due to treatment with X-rays.

THE IMMUNOFLUORESCENT TEST

This test which was pioneered by Burnham and Cormane should be able to provide an unequivocal answer as to whether a lesion is LE or not. It depends on the demonstration of immunoglobulin and complement bound to the basement membrane region of the epidermis. The globulin is detected by an immunofluorescence technique using fluorescein-tagged antihuman globulin. The fluorescein conjugate is incubated with cryostat sections from biopsies of the lesions in doubt, and resulting fluorescence at the site of bound globulin is recognized by fluorescence microscopy. A similar type of fluorescence can be demonstrated in lesions of pemphigoid but in this disease there are also circulating antibodies against the basement membrane area. In addition, the pattern of the immunofluorescent deposit differs in that it appears more 'tubular' than in discoid LE.

LABORATORY FINDINGS

It is not uncommon to find one or more of the following in patients with discoid LE without evidence of dissemination.
1. Raised ESR.
2. Leucopenia.
3. Raised level of serum gammaglobulin.
4. Positive antinuclear factor.
5. Positive Coombs' test (or positive DNA binding test).

The presence of one or more of these abnormalities in a patient with discoid LE should be regarded as an integral part of the disease and not necessarily a sign of systemic involvement.

HISTOPATHOLOGY

The histopathological features of this condition are:
1. Basal cell liquefaction degeneration.
2. Thickening of the basement membrane.
3. Irregular epidermal atrophy.
4. Relative hyperkeratosis.
5. Dermal oedema and focal connective tissue damage.
6. A closely applied perivascular infiltrate composed predominantly of lymphocytes in the mid and upper dermis and around the adnexal structures.
7. A variable degree of scarring and telangiectasia.

The typical changes are seen in *Fig.* 43.

The amount of basal cell damage is variable and on this feature depend the other epidermal changes seen. Occasionally the cellular infiltrate is more lichenoid, and in the presence of marked basal cell changes a picture is seen similar to atrophic lichen planus. The basal cell damage results in the release of melanin granules into the dermis, where some are engulfed by macrophages. The degree of melanin incontinence increases with increasing depth of skin pigmentation of the individual. A frequently overstressed feature is the presence of follicular plugging. The presence of horny plugs in follicles is so common in inflammatory dermatoses of the face that its presence cannot be used as a diagnostic pointer. In addition to the plugging of follicles by horn, the blocking of the eccrine sweat orifices may also be seen in discoid LE.

The lymphocytic perivascular cuffing may be similar to that seen in the figurate erythemas, but the lack of epidermal changes differentiate them from LE. The presence of a dense lymphocytic infiltrate around the upper and mid dermal blood vessels characterizes Jessner's lymphocytic infiltration of the skin. This can be mistaken for discoid LE, but the absence of the epidermal changes and the density of the infiltrate should enable a clear differentiation to be made.

Elastotic degeneration may be present to a greater degree than might be expected from the age or previous sun-exposure of the patient. In addition, other dermal changes may be seen, including dermal oedema and loss of elastic fibres in the involved areas; these may occur in any seriously inflammatory condition.

Areas of connective tissue damage may be observed, with loss of definition of connective tissue bundles and with changes in staining properties. Small areas of mucin deposition between connective tissue bundles can be distinguished by metachromatic stains, but the significance of this observation is entirely unknown. Scarring is a feature of most long-standing lesions together with destruction of appendages and telangiectasia. The blood vessels themselves are rarely markedly involved, although occasionally a degree of hyaline change may be seen in vessel walls.

LE Profundus

In this variant the epidermis may be unaffected. There is a striking patchy alteration in the connective tissue of the lower dermis and fat (Fountain, 1968). Areas are seen with loss of definition of connective tissue bundles and with increased eosinophia. These 'necrobiotic' foci seem to excite little change from the surrounding dermis. There is more involvement of small dermal blood vessels and, as in ordinary discoid LE, they are richly endowed with surrounding lymphocytes.

DIFFERENTIAL DIAGNOSIS

Discoid LE is diagnosed without difficulty in the presence of advanced scarred lesions, but difficulties arise when there are small early lesions or when a solitary reddened patch is present.

1. *Solar keratosis.* A well-defined pink scaly area on the cheek or forehead measuring up to 1 cm in diameter cannot be clinically diagnosed with confidence and histological arbitration may be required.

2. *Jessner's lymphocytic infiltration.* There are no epidermal changes in this condition and the lesions are either papular or plaque-like. In addition, lesions may also be present over the upper trunk and the lesions may be transient.

3. *Eczematous* conditions do not usually have well-defined borders and are not scarred or atrophic. Eczema is usually itchy and may be oozy or crusted.

4. *Lupus vulgaris* is now extremely rare and is unlikely to be a cause of serious practical difficulty for differential diagnosis. It is more granulomatous in appearance and often causes more destruction than discoid LE.

5. *Rosacea.* Patches of turgid erythema affecting just one cheek, or perhaps one cheek and the chin, can be mistaken for discoid LE. The presence of papules and pustules and indistinct margins favour rosacea.

6. *Superficial pemphigus.* Scaling and crusted patches which may persist are often seen without erosions or blisters in this type of pemphigus. Pemphigus foliaceus and pemphigus erythematosus differ only slightly, and the latter condition is so named because of its resemblance to LE. Coexistence of LE and pemphigus has been recorded by Chorzelski et al. (1968), so that the physical resemblance of the lesions may be more than a coincidence.

TREATMENT

Regrettably treatment is palliative and not curative.

1. Corticosteroids

Topical use of potent corticosteroids, particularly fluocinolone acetonide (Marsden, 1968), is sometimes helpful but is unpredictable and can lead to considerable atrophy. Occlusion with plastic film at night aids penetration of the lesion, and this can be used if ordinary application is ineffective. If the affected area is uneven (as it is more often than not on the face) then a plastic mould can be used to wear over the film at night. Some preparations containing greater than normal concentrations of the corticosteroids have been used—for example, fluocinolone acetonide 0·2 per cent—and these, it is claimed, are more effective in chronic discoid LE. Their use should be carefully supervised as considerable absorption of steroid can occur, and the problem of atrophy is even more pronounced than with the routine preparations.

Intradermal injections with triamcinolone acetonide suspensions or methyl prednisolone into the active edge of the lesion are sometimes successful. A modern method of administering this type of treatment is with one of the air 'jet' guns.

The use of systemic corticosteroids for this chronic persistent disease is permissible for rapidly progressive and destructive disease, but such use should be rare. Short courses may be helpful during these periods of activity and where lesions appear to be spreading, but should be avoided for the patient with two or three patches of chronic LE.

2. Antimalarials

Quinine was the first antimalarial of help in discoid LE. Later chloro-quine and mepacrine were found to have a therapeutic action as well (Gold, 1967). Chloroquine enjoyed a considerable vogue until 1966 or 1967. Its popularity rightly ended when the full potential of its toxicity was recognized. Copeman comprehensively reviewed the subject of chloroquine and discussed its toxicity fully (Copeman, 1967). Mild gastro-intestinal disturbances including nausea and abdominal dis-comfort are quite common with both chloroquine and mepacrine. Some haziness of vision and 'halo formation' may be experienced, resulting from chloroquine deposits in the cornea. Much more important and fortunately less common is an irreversible retinopathy which can lead to blindness. Mostly this tragic consequence has occurred in those patients on chloroquine for more than 1 year, and who have had doses of more than 400 mg per day. An early change seen on retinoscopy is the presence of pigmentation at the macula. Later a typical 'bull's eye' macular degeneration is seen. It has been claimed that the earliest detectable change is a differential loss of visual acuity for red light, and that at this stage the retinopathy is reversible.

Some clinicians maintain that chloroquine should now never be used for discoid LE in view of its dangers. There are others, however, who maintain that short courses (less than 3 months) on a dose of up to 400 mg per day may be justifiable where the disease is otherwise uncontrollable and the disease is producing considerable destruction and deformity.

3. Cryotherapy

The freezing of the advancing edge is a primitive but sometimes successful method for arresting the spread of a lesion. The usual method employed is the application of a freezing mixture of carbon dioxide snow and acetone with a cotton-wool swab to the advancing edge so that it turns white for a period of up to 1 minute. Severe blistering with pain and scar formation can result, so that some experience and guidance are necessary before the novice attempts this form of treatment.

4. Gold Salts

A course of calcium auriothiomalate injections, as for rheumatoid arthritis, used to be sometimes recommended, but it is doubtful whether its use ever produced substantial benefit, and it is infrequently em-ployed today. There is an impressive list of side-effects resulting from the use of gold injections including exfoliative dermatitis, lichenoid drug eruptions, nephrotic syndrome and aplastic anaemia.

5. Immunosuppressive Drugs

Both azathioprine and methotrexate have been used for systemic LE, but their use is not justifiable for discoid LE.

AETIOLOGY AND PATHOGENESIS

Lupus erythematosus is regarded as the archetypical auto-immune disease affecting many organ systems. However, the evidence for this is less than overwhelming. Fixed gammaglobulin and complement can be detected in the basement membrane zone at the site of lesions in discoid LE, and at both involved sites and in apparently unaffected skin in systemic LE. However, there are no detectable circulating antibodies to the basement membrane zone. Virtually all patients with systemic LE and about 35 per cent of those with discoid LE have a positive antinuclear factor test. What roles, if any, the fixed antibody at the basement membrane or the circulating antibody to DNA have in the pathogenesis of LE, or what interrelationships these two antibodies have, are entirely obscure. Van Joost (1973) demonstrated complement and immunoglobulin deposits in the junctional zone, but could find no DNA in the complexes.

The concept of this disorder having its basis in disordered immunity is supported by the ability of some drugs (notably hydralazine and procainamide) to provoke systemic LE.

Recently, however, cytoplasmic particles have been found electron microscopically in the lesions of both systemic and discoid LE that have been interpreted as viral in origin (Haustein, 1973). Even if they are later confirmed as virus particles, their role in LE will still be uncertain. Furthermore, even if it turns out that infection with these virus particles is the initiating event in this disorder, the pathogenesis of the lesions will still be basically auto-immune.

Sylvester et al. (1973) detected antibodies to double-stranded RNA in 42 per cent of discoid LE patients and in 70 per cent of those with systemic LE. This type of RNA is found only in trace amounts in normal skin, but is associated with viruses (particularly reo viruses) and with tissues infected with virus. This suggests that this RNA is exogenous in origin.

The relationship of this disorder to sunlight is also of considerable interest. It is obvious that the lesions are distributed predominantly on the light-exposed areas. In addition many patients relate that their lesions first appeared after a period of sun exposure or that their disease becomes active after being in the sun.

It has been shown that patients with LE have undue sensitivity in the sunburn region of the spectrum, and may develop patches of discoid LE at the site of testing (Epstein et al., 1965). Whether this is a specific response to sunlight or whether the lesions at the site of irradiation represent an isomorphic response to the injury caused by ultraviolet light is not entirely known. However, it is more likely that some specific response to ultraviolet light is involved, as some patients have developed flare-ups of their systemic disease after sun exposure. Tan and Stoughton (1969) believe that one possible explanation is that ultraviolet light alters DNA in the epidermis which 'leaks back' into the circulation exciting antibody formation. The antibodies, although formed to 'altered DNA', might also react with normal DNA and cause cell injury in this way. Davis et al. (1974) found that 27 per cent of patients with discoid LE have anti-DNA antibodies in the range normally associated with systemic LE. This suggests that discoid LE and systemic LE have strong similarities. Burch and Rowell (1970) believed that discoid LE and systemic LE are genetically distinct on the basis of epidemiological considerations.

SKIN MANIFESTATIONS OF SYSTEMIC LUPUS ERYTHEMATOSUS

Approximately 70 per cent of patients with systemic LE have some skin manifestations of the disease. Of these, one-third to one-half have the classical butterfly erythema affecting the cheeks and the nose (*Plate* 7B). The reddened areas are quite well delineated and may be swollen and oedematous looking. Patchy discoid erythema over the face, upper limbs and trunk is seen and these lesions may develop scaling and resemble discoid LE.

Subcutaneous nodules occur in 5 per cent of patients (Tuffanelli and Dubois, 1964). They are similar to rheumatoid nodules and the most frequently involved site is the extensor aspect of the forearm. Urticaria occurs in the surprisingly high proportion of 7 per cent. Raynaud's phenomenon, alopecia and ulcerations are other skin manifestations.

SKIN MANIFESTATIONS OF DERMATOMYOSITIS

This uncommon connective tissue disorder is briefly discussed here because it may present as an acute dermatosis of the face.

Classically the disease starts insidiously with muscle pain and weakness. At the same time, reddened areas start to appear symmetrically on the face, limbs and hands. On the hands the periungual tissues become reddened and a curious irregular hypertrophy of the cuticle is seen. Streaks of dusky erythema appear over the dorsa of the fingers and on the backs of the hands.

The temples and malar regions also become reddened and swollen. The colour is characteristic and has a mauve or lilac hue. The upper face, and particularly the periorbital regions, may become very swollen and may fox the inexperienced into diagnosing angioneurotic oedema (*Fig.* 44).

REFERENCES

Burch P. R. J. and Rowell N. R. (1970) Lupus erythematosus. Analysis of the sex— and age—distributions of the discoid and systemic forms of the disease in different countries. *Acta Derm. Venereol. (Stockh.)* **50**, 293.

Chorzelski T., Jablonska S. and Blaszczyk M. (1968) Immunopathological investigations in the Senear–Usher syndrome (co-existence of pemphigus and lupus erythematosus). *Br. J. Dermatol.* **80**, 211.

Copeman P. W. (1967) Chloroquine. *Trans. St John's Hosp. Dermatol. Soc.* **53**, 24.

Davis P., Atkins B. and Hughes G. R. V. (1974) Antibodies to native DNA in discoid lupus erythematosus. *Br. J. Dermatol.* **91**, 175.

Epstein J. H. and Tuffanelli D. L. (1966) Discoid lupus erythematosus. In: Dubois, E. L. (ed.) *Lupus Erythematosus.* New York, McGraw-Hill.

Epstein J. H., Tuffanelli D. L. and Dubois E. L. (1965) Light sensitivity and lupus erythematosus. *Arch. Dermatol.* **91**, 483.

Fountain R. B. (1968) Lupus erythematosus profundus. *Br. J. Dermatol.* **80**, 571.

Gold S. C. (1960) Progress in the understanding of lupus erythematosus. *Br. J. Dermatol.* **72**, 231.

Gold S. C. (1967) Management of cutaneous lupus erythematosus. *Br. Med. J.* **1**, 224.

Haustein U. F. (1973) Tubular structures in affected and normal skin in chronic discoid and systemic lupus erythematosus. Electron microscopic studies. *Br. J. Dermatol.* **89**, 1.

Klemperer P., Pollack A. D. and Baehr G. (1941) Pathology of disseminated lupus erythematosus. *Arch. Pathol.* **32**, 569.

Lodin A. and Thyresson N. (1955) Discoid and disseminated lupus erythematosus. *Acta Derm. Venereol. (Stockh.)* **35**, 429.

Marsden C. W. (1968) Fluocinolone acetonide 0·2% cream. A co-operative clinical trial. *Br. J. Dermatol.* **80**, 614.

Sylvester R. A., Attias M., Talal N. and Tuffanelli D. L. (1973) Antibodies to viral and synthetic double stranded RNA in discoid lupus erythematosus. *Arthritis Rheumatol.* **16**, 383.

Tan E. M. and Stoughton R. B. (1969) Ultra violet light induced damage to desoxyribonucleic acid in human skin. *J. Invest. Dermatol.* **52**, 537.

Tuffanelli D. L. and Dubois E. L. (1964) Cutaneous manifestations of systemic lupus erythematosus. *Arch. Dermatol.* **90**, 377.

Van Joost J. (1973) An attempt to identify the nature of immunoglobulins—complement deposits in the skin in lupus erythematosus. *Br. J. Dermatol.* **89**, 15.

Chapter 7

The Face and Sunlight

INTRODUCTION

Undoubtedly we would be better off retaining the Victorian standards of feminine allure by admiring women who are pale and 'interesting'. Modern sun worship has both short-term and long-term drawbacks. This chapter briefly considers the facial disorders caused, precipitated or aggravated by the sun. The areas predominantly affected are the forehead, the cheeks, the point of the chin and the nose. In bald men the pate is at risk and in both sexes the ears are affected according to the degree of cover afforded by the current fashion in hair styles. The lower neck is often involved. Areas that are conspicuously spared in photodermatoses are those in the 'shade', i.e. the hairy scalp, behind the ears and just under the chin. The margin between involved and uninvolved skin may not be as sharp as expected and depends on the particular disorder.

Sunlight-produced rashes mostly start to occur during the spring and summer months. There are several notable exceptions—Hutchinson's summer prurigo and polymorphic light eruption, for example, which may make their appearance annually in February. There are two aspects to the problem of where and when the photodermatoses occur—firstly the stimulus, and secondly the biological status of the stimulated tissue.

The Stimulus to Photodermatoses

Harmful effects from solar irradiation are confined to the ultraviolet light area in the electromagnetic spectrum—that is radiation between 250 and 410 nanometres. For all intents and purposes visible light is harmless. It is usually a small portion of the ultraviolet light zone in the spectrum that is to blame—maybe even a single 'waveband', for example 'the Soret band' (410 nm) in porphyria. The relevant spectrum for a particular disease is known as the action spectrum and may be determined in irradiating the skin with a monochromatic source of light ('a monochromator'). The development of a photodermatosis is to some extent dependent on the total energy of the relevant radiation received by the light-sensitive tissue. The amount of energy received depends on (*a*) the angle at which the sun's rays are received, i.e. the latitude and the time of the day, (*b*) the intensity which is dependent on the altitude and the amount of cloud cover, and (*c*) the length of the exposure.

It is possible to receive harmful ultraviolet radiation from artificial sources. The obvious examples are lamps that are specifically designed to emit ultraviolet light. However, there are less obvious sources, including the ordinary domestic or office fluorescent tube form of lighting, which may be of importance in some clinical situations. It should be noted that most window glass filters out radiation below 400 nm (allowing the Soret band through), but certain types of window glass allow some ultraviolet light through.

Biological Status of Stimulated Tissue

All other things being equal, the amount of injury experienced by normal tissue is proportional to the amount of photoprotection afforded by the degree of pigmentation. The more pigmentation possessed by the individual the less likely are short-term and long-term sequelae from solar exposure. There are also inherited biochemical faults which lead to enhanced reactivity or increased injury of the irradiated tissue (e.g. porphyria and xeroderma pigmentosum—*see below*). The environment may also lead to enhanced reactivity or increased injury. Thus, either the application (intentional or otherwise) of certain chemicals to the skin or the ingestion of others can result in a specific hypersensitivity or in a non-specific toxic reaction (photo-allergy and phototoxicity).

Sunburn

Most of us have yearned for the healthy, bronzed outdoor look, sunbathed injudiciously and experienced the unpleasant temporary soreness of sunburn. The areas on the face that are worst affected are the forehead, the tops of the ears and bridge of the nose, though the cheeks may also suffer. In bald men the 'bald patch' is often severely affected. Soreness and redness are usually experienced within a few hours of exposure and these may persist for several days. After a period of 6–10 days desquamation begins. The reaction is severe in fair-haired, blue-eyed, light-complexioned individuals and especially in red-haired subjects with a 'ruddy' complexion (some Celtic types).

'Short-wave' ultraviolet light is responsible for this sunburn reaction. The wavelengths involved are 290–320 nm u.v.b.

In those who are particularly sensitive and have had a hefty dose of sunshine, the affected areas may become swollen and very painful.

Pigmentation may be accomplished without too much trauma by gradually increasing the exposure time. How this accommodation takes place is uncertain, but it seems to involve some epidermal hyperplasia.

The *pathology* of sunburn is interesting. Scattered throughout the affected epidermis are damaged cells which are eosinophilic, swollen and homogenized—'sunburn cells' (*Fig.* 45). The cause of the persistent erythema may be the release of prostaglandins and can be reduced by drugs that inhibit prostaglandin synthetase—the enzyme that synthesizes these mediator materials. Prevention is far easier than cure and if the subject cannot be dissuaded from risking 'Apollo's wrath', he or she should use an efficient light screen on the areas to be exposed immediately prior to the exposure. The best are those that are based on para-amino benzoic acid. Reapplication after 1–2 hours is usually necessary—especially after swimming.

Treatment

Aspirin administration may help and together with the application of topical corticosteroids is best reserved for severe cases.

LONG-TERM HAZARDS OF LIGHT EXPOSURE

Development of Skin Cancers

South Africa, Australia and the southern United States are countries that have, on the one hand, a hot sunny climate and, on the other, a population that is, at least in part, white-skinned and fair in complexion. In these countries the treatment of small cutaneous malignancies forms a major part of dermatological practice. The relationship between sun exposure and the development of cutaneous neoplasms is now well established (Urbach, 1969). Those mainly at risk are individuals with fair skin and blue eyes. Some Celtic groups seem to have the propensity for the development of skin cancers even though they have a darker complexion. The particular neoplasms that occur frequently are solar keratoses (which are 'premalignant' lesions—*see* Chapter 9), basal cell and squamous cell epitheliomata (*see* Chapter 9), kerato-acanthomata (*see* Chapter 9), and to a lesser extent malignant melanomata (*see* Chapter 9).

The length of exposure necessary before serious and irreversible damage has been done is difficult to know, because there are so many factors that have to be taken into account including pigmentation and intensity of exposure.

Solar (Senile) Elastosis

This is a specific degenerative change in dermal connective tissue due to exposure to solar irradiation. There are characteristic histological changes (*Fig.* 46) in the upper and papillary dermis. Immediately below the epidermis there is a narrow band of normal connective tissue; beneath this normal zone there is more basophilic material that is either arranged in 'chunky wavy fibres' (resembling 'chopped spaghetti') or in homogenized glassy areas. This change may not be seen in every dermal papilla when the degree of 'elastosis' is minimal or may involve every papilla and extend into the mid dermis when there is a severe degree of degeneration. The term 'elastosis' is descriptive of the staining properties as the material stains brown or black with orcein. It does not imply that the material necessarily *is* elastic tissue. There has been considerable debate as to what the altered connective tissue actually consists of and it seems that there is moderately good evidence that it is more like collagen than elastin. The subject was well reviewed by Mitchell Sams and Graham Smith (1965). Elastotic degeneration is not specific to ultraviolet light irradiation and is frequently observed after X-ray treatment to the skin for cutaneous malignancies. It is also seen in areas that have been exposed to radiant heat (e.g. on the shins from coal fires) over a protracted period of time.

The clinical effects of elastotic degeneration are as follows:

1. The development of wrinkles, lines and crow's feet. The deep rhomboidal fissures seen at the back of the neck in elderly men who have been employed in outdoor jobs most of their lives ('sailor's neck').
2. A thickening and 'leathery' appearance of the skin.
3. The development of telangiectasia over the cheeks.
4. The development of large comedones periorbitally.

Presumably, the telangiectasia results from loss of support for vessels of the subpapillary venous plexus and the comedones that occur may be caused by the loss of follicular support by the dermal connective tissue framework. Not all facial lines and wrinkles are the result of elastotic degeneration. Dystrophic changes in dermal connective tissue due to weathering may be partially responsible and the loss of elasticity and thinning out of connective tissues with increasing age probably play some part in the development of wrinkles. It must also be said that biopsies of the face which show solar elastosis do not necessarily come from wrinkled or leathery areas.

Treatment
There is no effective treatment available.

GENETICALLY DETERMINED ABNORMAL REACTIONS TO LIGHT: PORPHYRIAS

In these disorders there are abnormalities in the synthetic pathways of the tetrapyrrole moiety of haem compounds.

Erythropoietic Protoporphyria (EPP)

Protoporphyrin occurs to excess in the red cells in this disease which is inherited as an autosomal dominant trait. It has only been recognized in the past 15 years or so (Magnus et al., 1961). It is quite uncommon but by no means rare.

Clinical Appearance

It sometimes presents in early infancy but is more commonly diagnosed first in childhood. Characteristically the sites that have been exposed to the sun feel uncomfortable and sore and become swollen and red a short time afterwards (about half an hour). The discomfort may cause considerable distress and before the disease was recognized many of these patients were labelled as neurotics. After some years the affected areas—particularly the bridge of the nose, the malar regions and the forehead—develop a thickened appearance and small pitted or pock-type scars are seen. Some patients with this disease were mistakenly diagnosed as having lipoid proteinosis—another rare but unrelated metabolic disorder. Apart from the dermatological complaint, patients with EPP may have systemic symptoms from pigment stones in the gall bladder and patients have also been described recently with cirrhosis of the liver as a complication.

Erythropoietic Porphyria (Günter's Disease)

This is an extremely rare congenitally determined fault in porphyrin synthesis. It causes a bullous destructive dermatosis of the light-exposed areas. In addition, the teeth are deformed, reddened and discoloured. There is facial hirsuties. The urine, which may be red, fluoresces red in ultraviolet light as do the teeth and the bones.

Porphyria Cutanea Tarda (PCT)

There are two kinds of PCT; both are uncommon. The first is known as *variegate porphyria* and occurs in families. The mode of inheritance appears to be dominant. There is a high incidence of this particular disorder in South Africa (Dean, 1963). The other variety is *'acquired' porphyria cutanea tarda* although this may also have a genetic basis. The cutaneous component of both is identical. The diseases differ in that in variegate porphyria (dominantly inherited) there is a systemic aspect to the disease identical to that of acute intermittent porphyria. Most patients with acquired porphyria cutanea tarda are chronic alcoholics although the condition has also been described as a result of a hepatoma. Other hepatotoxins have been incriminated, including hexachloro-benzene and chlorinated hydrocarbons. Barbiturates, sulphonamides and certain other drugs are known to provoke attacks of porphyria in those who are predisposed. Griseofulvin, chloroquine and oestrogens are other compounds that precipitate porphyric attacks.

Acquired Porphyria Cutanea Tarda. The light-exposed areas develop bullae and erosions after sun exposure, although the time interval varies. Milia occur at the affected sites later. The exposed areas are also more fragile and are very easily injured. These sites also develop prominent terminal hairs and become rather characteristically suffused and pigmented (*Fig.* 47). In some patients the skin becomes thickened and bound down in the light-exposed sites. This 'pseudosclerodermatous' condition is often misdiagnosed.

Treatment

Treatment of the underlying liver disease is obviously important and attention to any alcoholic habits is a prime necessity. Avoidance of the particularly harmful drugs is also necessary and where possible no drugs should be given at all, as many others are known which are potentially harmful. Avoidance of sun exposure is also important. It should be noted that porphyric patients are sensitive to the 'Soret band' in the spectrum (410 nm) which is transmitted by some types of window glass. The most useful form of therapy for porphyria cutanea tarda is venesection—weekly removal of 1 pint for perhaps 12 weeks has been recommended (Ramsay et al., 1974).

DRUG-INDUCED PHOTOSENSITIVITY

A number of drugs 'sensitize' the skin to the action of ultraviolet light. The commonest are the sulphonamides and the reaction that they cause may be very fierce (*Plate* 8A). It may be eczematous or erythematous. The tetracyclines are also photosensitizers and the worst offender in this regard appears to be demethylchlortetracycline. A curious form of light-induced nail disorder has been described under the influence of the tetracyclines (photo-onycholysis). The cutaneous disorder is usually a marked erythematous reaction. Nalidixic acid has been found to cause bullae on the skin after sun exposure and bullae may continue to appear some time after this drug has been stopped. Chlorpromazine in very high doses over long periods causes a curious reaction in which a purplish pigment is deposited in the light-exposed areas, producing 'purple people'.

PHOTOCONTACT REACTIONS

A number of substances when placed on the skin heighten the reactivity to incident ultraviolet light. They include the psoralens whose effects are utilized therapeutically and the similar furocoumarins which cause a 'phytophotodermatitis'. The halogenated salicylanilides are also well-known photosensitizers and were the cause of the light-sensitive dermatitis seen in the early 1960's due to these compounds being added to soaps as antiseptic agents. A number of naturally occurring oils and plant extracts cause photosensitization.

MISCELLANEOUS LIGHT REACTIONS

Polymorphic Light Eruption

This is a photodermatosis of unknown cause that seems to be constitutional in origin. The eruption which occurs in the light-exposed areas and in adjacent skin is either eczematous, nodular or plaque-like. It characteristically affects young women but other groups are not exempt. It recurs each year and may start in February when the increase in incident ultraviolet light is not generally noticeable.

Hutchinson's Summer Prurigo

This is another light-provoked dermatosis of unknown cause. The disorder affects younger age groups than polymorphic light eruption and there seems to be some kind of a genetic basis for its occurrence (Meara et al., 1971). The eruption it causes may closely resemble excoriated atopic dermatitis affecting the face and the backs of the hands and forearms (*Fig.* 48). It persists for many years and then may spontaneously remit. It is quite a disabling disorder and seems very refractory to most currently used anti-inflammatory topical treatments.

Jessner's Lymphocytic Infiltration of the Skin

The subject of cutaneous lymphocytic infiltrates is a thorny one for dermatologists and pathologists, but this disorder can be separated and defined more easily than most other conditions, which may share a few of its features. It has resemblances to discoid lupus erythematosus—especially histopathologically. The condition is characterized clinically by the development of pink or red hemispherical non-tender papules and plaques over the temples, cheeks, neck and shoulders (*Plate* 8B). Histologically there are 'clumps' and aggregates of small lymphocytes around the small blood vessels of the upper and mid dermis. The disorder affects both sexes and has a less easily defined relationship to solar exposure than many of the disorders already discussed. It lasts a variable period (recurring each summer time) and seems unassociated with any systemic component of lupus erythematosus. Application of potent topical corticosteroids appears to be marginally helpful in controlling the individual lesions.

Actinic Reticuloid

This condition is now established as a clinical entity. It was described by Ive et al. (1969) but may not be a 'new disease'. It characteristically affects middle-aged or elderly men. The eruption which is essentially a type of lichenified eczema is not restricted to the light-exposed areas but 'overflows' on to such sites as the palms and the trunk. Clinically, there is a very pronounced increase in skin markings or 'lichenification' (*Fig.* 49). This may be gross over the back of the neck or on the forehead. In addition, there may be a pigmentary anomaly—especially on the trunk. The disease is progressive and incapacitating. Patients with it appear to be hypersensitive to a wide band of wavelengths—in fact right into the visible part of the spectrum. They seem so exquisitely sensitive that even the light from domestic fluorescent light fittings is sufficient to keep the process going. Consequently, these patients should be nursed in a shaded room with a dimmed tungsten filament electric light. The usual topical anti-inflammatory measures are only slightly helpful. Histopathologically, there is an eczematous reaction affecting the epidermis and a variable amount of dermal inflammatory cell infiltrate. At times this infiltrate is so intense that the appearance is suggestive of a reticulosis—and this is how the name of 'reticuloid' arose. Systemic steroids and antimitotic agents have not been very successful.

Solar Urticaria

This is a rare form of 'physical urticaria'. The urticarial weals appear a variable time after exposure, but may be experienced after a few seconds. The 'exciting wavelength' varies in the individual patient. It is said that patients may be helped by desensitization by increasing lengths of exposure.

CONDITIONS AGGRAVATED BY LIGHT EXPOSURE

In this category can be included such conditions as rosacea, lupus erythematosus and some patients with atopic dermatitis. The exact reason for the exacerbating effect of light is unknown in each of these diseases. Indeed it may not be ultraviolet irradiation that is itself responsible, but rather associated stimuli. The effect of light in these conditions is not entirely predictable (even in the individual patient whose previous response is well known).

REFERENCES

Dean G. (1963) *The Porphyrias*. London, Pitman Medical.
Ive F. A., Magnus I. A., Warin R. P. and Wilson-Jones E. (1969) 'Actinic reticuloid.' A chronic dermatosis associated with severe photosensitivity and the histological resemblance to lymphoma. *Br. J. Dermatol.* **81**, 469.

Magnus I. A., Jarrett A., Prankerd T. A. J. and Rimington C. (1961) Erythropoietic protoporphyria. A new porphyrin syndrome with solar urticaria due to protoporphyrinaemia. *Lancet* **11**, 448.

Meara R. H., Magnus I. A., Grice K., Wilson-Jones E. and Johansson S. G. O. (1971) Hutchinson's summer prurigo. *Trans. St John's Hosp. Dermatol. Soc.* **57**, 87.

Mitchell Sams W., jun. and Graham Smith J., jun. (1965) Alterations in human dermal fibrous connective tissue with age and chronic sun damage. In: Montagna, W. (ed.) *Advances in Biology of the Skin*, Vol. 6, Aging. Oxford, Pergamon, p. 199.

Ramsay C. A., Magnus I. A., Turnbull A. and Baker H. (1974) The treatment of porphyria cutanea tarda by venesection. *Q. J. Med.* **43**, 1.

Urbach F. (ed.) (1969) *The Biological Effects of Ultra Violet Radiation.* Oxford, Pergamon.

Chapter 8

Infections of the Skin of the Face

BACTERIAL

1. Impetigo

This is predominantly an infection of children, although young adults are also sometimes affected. It is more common in socially deprived groups. It was quite frequent before, during and just after the 1939–45 War, but became much less common in the 1950's and the first half of the 1960's. In recent years it seems to be once again more frequently seen.

The clinical picture is quite distinctive although it is only too often misdiagnosed. The face is one of the most commonly involved sites but the infection may be seen on the trunk or limbs as well, especially in babies. The affected site is first reddened then rapidly becomes moist and develops a characteristic honey-coloured crust (*Fig.* 50). Sometimes blisters are the first sign of the infection and they appear to arise from an inflamed area so that to the inexperienced the bullous variety presents a diagnostic problem. It has been suggested that these blisters are more likely to occur if the impetigo is mistakenly treated with topical corticosteroids at the outset.

The natural history of the disorder, if left untreated, is that individual involved areas eventually heal but new ones continue to appear for some months. When the lesions do heal the areas stay a dusky-red colour for some weeks afterwards before finally fading.

Differential Diagnosis

In differential diagnosis the following should be considered:

a. Seborrhoeic Dermatitis/Infectious Eczematoid Dermatitis. There is a variety of eczema that occurs in well-defined discoid and irregular patches that becomes exudative and crusted, and which may be difficult to distinguish from true impetigo. When this rash becomes crusted it is often referred to as 'impetiginized' although bacteriologically this is probably a misnomer.

Certainly adequate treatment with topical steroids alone is sufficient to clear this type of eczema without the addition of antibiotics or other antimicrobial compounds (Davies et al., 1968).

b. Pemphigus Foliaceus. Persistent oozy, scaling and crusted patches on the face and trunk are also characteristic of this acantholytic disorder. These lesions do not clear with anti-impetigo treatment, tend to occur in an older age group than does impetigo and usually do not possess the characteristic golden crust of impetigo. Biopsy should theoretically distinguish pemphigus but in practice this may be difficult, especially if the epidermal 'split' is an extremely high one. The immunofluorescence tests— direct and indirect (Beutner et al., 1970)—are probably more reliable.

c. Herpes Simplex. When the vesicles that characterize this condition burst, a crust often forms and then the condition may resemble impetigo, but the history of recurrent attacks precipitated by a pyrexial illness or some other easily detected stimulus should help distinguish the two. Herpes spontaneously clears in 7-12 days but impetigo tends to persist.

Bacteriology

There has been some confusion in the literature between impetigo and other types of pyoderma. Some workers have extended their understanding of the term 'impetigo' to cover most cutaneous pyodermas. This may explain some of the reports suggesting that the haemolytic streptococcus is the most important causative organism. The reports of Kaplan et al. (1970) on the epidemic impetigo and glomerulonephritis in the Red Lake Indians and likewise the reports of Poon-King et al. (1967) on the same situation in the West Indies describe what is probably an ecthymatous pyoderma rather than the more superficial impetigo seen in the United Kingdom.

A recent investigation (Connor, 1972) has established that in the type of impetigo seen in this country both the haemolytic streptococcus and *Staphylococcus aureus* may be isolated from the majority of lesions. They found that they could isolate both micro-organisms in 18 per cent of their patients; beta-haemolytic streptococci were isolated alone in 21 per cent and *Staphylococcus aureus* in 87 per cent.

Undoubtedly acute glomerulonephritis can follow streptococcal infection of the skin. It seems that this happens much more frequently in some epidemics of skin infection than in others. Those associated with nephritis are caused by nephritogenic strains of streptococci. However, this complication does not often seem to follow the superficial type of impetigo contagiosa seen in the United Kingdom.

Treatment

In cases where the infection is not limited to a very small area, the best treatment is with a systemic antibiotic, and penicillin is most suitable unless contraindicated by the patient's hypersensitivity or by the known presence of resistant micro-organisms. For very limited infections topical therapy is permissible. Crusts should be washed gently away with a detergent antiseptic solution such as 1 per cent aqueous Cetavlon and an antibacterial application used two or three times per day. A hydroxyquinoline such as Vioform may be used. Topical antibiotics are not recommended as they may sensitize the patient or, if of low sensitizing potential, either they are inappropriate because they are used systemically or they have the wrong spectrum of antibacterial activity. The condition is contagious and until the child is free of crusts he should not be allowed to attend school or play with other children. Treatment is usually effective in 7–10 days.

2. Erysipelas

This used to be more common than it is today and was, in addition, a serious and sometimes fatal disease. The lower leg is probably the area most frequently involved but the face—particularly the cheeks and forehead—is also a common site for erysipelas.

Characteristically it is of sudden onset with fever, malaise and tenderness in the affected areas. Shortly afterwards the local signs become more evident with swelling and redness (*Plate* 9A). The site may be quite sharply defined with an obviously advancing edge. There is often a purpuric component to the redness and the surface of the involved skin may also show vesiculation (particularly at the margins). As the cheeks may be involved and there is redness, this condition is sometimes mistaken for rosacea. However, the cheeks are hot and tender in erysipelas, the patient is ill and the history is short. These points should serve to distinguish the conditions easily. Erysipelas should also not be confused with recurrent cellulitis of the face, in which there is usually the story of a series of attacks of swelling and pain occurring diffusely over an area of the face. In between attacks the swelling persists to some extent. The colour of the affected area is a deeper red and less purpuric. In addition there is a less well-defined edge to the affected area. Altogether erysipelas of the face is a more acute and more serious illness.

Histologically there is a surprising amount of oedema present sub-epidermally and there is a considerable amount of bleeding present as well (*Fig.* 51). Attempts at culturing a micro-organism are rarely successful in the author's experience. The causative organism is reputedly a haemolytic streptococcus but for some reason it appears to be very difficult to isolate.

Treatment

The most suitable treatment is with antibiotics and the antibiotic of choice is penicillin. A 5-day course starting with 500 mg by mouth of phenoxymethyl penicillin and continuing with 250 mg 6-hourly is usually adequate. When there is a history of penicillin sensitivity, erythromycin is indicated.

3. Cellulitis of the Face

This is a clinical entity but it is doubtful whether it is due to a single causative agent.

It is characterized by recurrent attacks of pain and swelling in an area of the face accompanied by malaise and fever. In between attacks, which usually last 2–7 days, there is a persistent puffy area at the site of the infection. The areas most frequently involved are the sides of the nose and the medial portions of the cheeks, but the upper lip and forehead can also be affected in this way. Eventually the area becomes perpetually grossly swollen and almost indistinguishable from the chronic lymphoedema seen in rosacea.

Aetiology

Although it is often presumed that pathogenic bacteria gain entry through 'cracks around the nose' there rarely appears to be any clinical evidence for this concept.

Pathology

In between acute episodes the involved area shows dermal oedema, dilated small vessels and a variable number of lymphohistiocytic cells but no specific changes.

Treatment

Antibiotics are indicated and the ones usually prescribed are those that are empirically found to be most effective and free of side-effects in the particular patient. Tetracyclines are frequently prescribed particularly if some type of prophylactic and long-term administration is indicated.

4. Sycosis Barbae

This is a persistent and troublesome folliculitis of the beard area in men.

It is frequently called 'shaving rash'. As with other bacterial infections it is much less common than it used to be, although a mild form is still quite often seen. Clinically it is a papular and papulo-pustular eruption of the beard area, and the majority of the lesions are follicular in origin. If severe it can produce an oozing painful inflammatory dermatosis of the face. This condition must be distinguished from ingrowing hairs (pili recurvati) in which hairs emerge from their follicles at an acute angle, and because of their natural curvature repenetrate the skin causing inflammatory papules.

Bacteriology
The condition does not appear to be caused by a specific single or group of micro-organisms. However, very little is known of the bacteriology and this view might later have to be altered.

Treatment
A prolonged course of penicillin (250 mg 6-hourly for 2 weeks) together with a change of shaving habit is usually sufficient. Thus a change to an electric razor can be very helpful. Resolution also appears to be helped by the application of a weak corticosteroid such as hydrocortisone (preferably in a cream base), and the use of a non-irritant detergent antiseptic such as 1 per cent aqueous Cetavlon.

Tuberculosis and the Face

1. *Lupus Vulgaris*
See Chapter 10.

2. *Tuberculous Sinuses in the Neck*
These are still occasionally seen originating from underlying tuberculous lymphadenitis.

3. '*Tuberculids*'
Acne agminata and rosaceous tuberculid of Lewandowski are no longer thought of as hypersensitivity phenomena to tuberculosis elsewhere.

Leprosy

Lepromatous leprosy involves the face in a rather characteristic way giving rise to 'leonine facies'. The possibility of the diagnosis frequently comes up when a granulomatous biopsy from the skin of the face is discussed but more detailed treatment is outside the scope of this book.

VIRAL INFECTIONS OF THE SKIN

1. Viral Warts

These common benign epithelial proliferations are of two morphological patterns on the face—plane warts which are the most frequent, and 'common warts'. Sometimes the verrucous surface of common warts is exaggerated to give a filiform pattern and such lesions seem more common around the nose, lips and on the scalp. Viral warts are caused by a small DNA virus of the 'polyoma' group. The wart virus has a crystalline pattern of an icosahedron and the characteristic pattern of the virus may be seen electron microscopically in a comparatively simple test employing phosphotungstic acid staining of curetted wart material (Kingsley-Smith et al., 1967). Mention is made of this investigation as it enables a rapid distinction to be made between viral warts and other epithelial nodules. Their infectivity seems to be low but very little is known of their epidemiology. These lesions are most common in children but are by no means confined to them. They are also seen on the face of young adults, especially men in whom they may be troublesome on the beard area where they may occur in great numbers.

Histologically there is epithelial proliferation with acanthosis and papillomatosis. Sometimes a characteristic vacuolation is seen in cells infected with wart virus. In addition, infected cells may show basophilic inclusions in the cytoplasm which probably represent altered keratin and smaller intranuclear eosinophilic inclusions that may represent viral aggregates.

Differential Diagnosis

This should include mollusca contagiosa, seborrhoeic keratoses, actinic keratoses, kerato-acanthomata and squamous cell carcinomata. Occasionally the lesions are so prolific as to simulate a dermatosis (*Plate* 9B).

Treatment

This should be resisted if possible as most lesions spontaneously regress after a variable period (*Lancet*, 1974).

Vigorous treatment of these lesions is probably never justified in young children and the most active preparation that the author uses on the face is salicylic acid collodion (BPC). Often one of the coloured dyes (such as gentian violet) is the most appropriate treatment. Where large numbers of warts occur around the neck, and elsewhere on the beard area in adults, light cautery is permissible if other measures fail.

2. Molluscum Contagiosum

These lesions are also benign epithelial proliferations and are also caused by a virus. The virus in the case of this condition is a large RNA virus belonging to the 'pox group' (which also includes smallpox and vaccinia virus). The commonest sites for these lesions are the moist intertriginous zones and the face, but virtually anywhere may be involved. They are seen not infrequently around the mouth, around the eyelids (where they can give rise to diagnostic difficulty) and on the forehead.

Clinical Appearance. The lesions are umbilicated globular nodules 1–5 mm in diameter and grey or creamy white in colour. In fact, they have a wide range of clinical appearance and they are often misdiagnosed. Approximately 10 per cent of mollusca have an associated inflammatory component (De Oreo et al., 1956). Often this takes the form of a reddened halo around the nodule—sometimes this component is more frankly eczematous and may not be arranged symmetrically around the molluscum. In this latter instance there is a real difficulty in knowing whether the viral lesions gave rise to the mollusca or an eczematous process predisposed to the viral infection. Certainly both mollusca and viral warts appear to be more common in atopic dermatitis.

Giant molluscum lesions around the eyes may simulate basal cell epitheliomata and when the lesions are minute and present in large numbers they may be mistaken for a dermatosis.

Histology. Molluscum contagiosum consists of an area of epidermal thickening which is undergoing a characteristic degenerative change most pronounced at the surface. The cells form eosinophilic globular 'molluscum bodies within their cytoplasm' which are discharged at the surface (*Fig.* 52).

Treatment

The traditional method of puncturing the molluscum with an orange stick dipped in liquor phenolis is not to be encouraged. They are equally well treated by squeezing out the curd-like contents with forceps or by briefly applying the electrocautery to each lesion.

3. Herpes Simplex

The herpes simplex virus is one of the smallest human viruses and is in the same group as the chickenpox virus. There are two antigenic strains, HSV.1 and HSV.2. The second one has been found to be associated with genital herpes only and will not be further considered here (recently its role in cervical carcinoma has been discussed— *British Medical Journal*, 1972).

Clinical Appearance. Two main types of disease are produced by herpes simplex, dependent on the immune status of the infected individual. The first type is primary herpes simplex and is seen in individuals who have had no previous experience of the infection. Generally this takes the form of a mild pyrexial illness with a stomatitis or pharyngitis. Occasionally a very much more severe generalized illness results in which hepatitis or a meningo-encephalitis is seen and which may have a fatal outcome. A widespread infection of the skin may also be seen as part of this 'primary disease'.

Disseminated cutaneous involvement may also arise as a complication of atopic dermatitis or more rarely other dermatoses including Darier's disease and seborrhoeic dermatitis. A severe and widespread herpes infection may also be seen in patients being treated with cytotoxic agents and corticosteroids and those with either congenital or acquired diseases of the immune system.

The best known clinical sign of herpes simplex infection is the 'cold sore'. This common and annoying disorder appears to be the result of an unusual biological mechanism in which some precipitating event causes the virus to migrate to the skin from the trigeminal ganglion, where it probably normally resides (Bastian et al., 1972; Baringer and Swoveland, 1973). In recurrent cold sores this sequence is repeated at quite frequent intervals. The precipitating agent may be readily identifiable and quite trivial, such as the premenstrual period or a slight rise in body temperature. The affected subject has circulating antibodies to the herpes virus and recurrent attacks of cold sores are not a manifestation of disordered immune mechanisms.

The lesions of recurrent herpes simplex usually occur around the mouth (*Fig.* 53) or nose but may be seen elsewhere on the face and are occasionally seen on areas of the body such as the buttock or penis. The usual sequence of events is as follows: The involved area becomes raised and reddened; then after 2–3 days discrete vesicles form. These may become turbid and pustular before a final stage after 6–10 days when crusts form which eventually drop off leaving a pink unscarred area. Attacks may only occur during a high fever in some individuals but in other more unfortunate patients clusters of lesions may reappear as frequently as once a month.

A further precipitating factor besides the premenstrual period and fever is exposure to the sun.

Diagnosis

1. The clinical diagnosis can be confirmed by finding the typical degenerate epithelial cells on a smear from the lesions. The cells are large with pale pink cytoplasm and dark pyknotic nuclei, multi-nucleate cells may also be seen. The cells are rounded, having lost their intercellular contacts.

2. A more specific investigation is an immunofluorescent test in which a smear from a lesion is treated with an antiherpes serum conjugated with fluorescein isothiocyanate. This is a rapid and useful test and is specific for herpes.

3. Biopsy will reveal characteristic reticular degeneration within the epidermis leading to vesicle formation.

4. Viral culture on chick chorio-allantoic membrane can be performed where there is a virological department at hand.

Treatment

Repeated vaccination is ineffectual and founded on the two false premises that vaccinia and herpes simplex have common antigenic determinants and that there is a deficiency in the level of circulating antibodies to herpes simplex. The only treatment that has been found of any value is the topical use of idoxuridine (5-IDU), an antiviral compound, which is an RNA inhibitor. This has been found useful when given by a jet injector, and when applied topically in dimethyl sulphoxide at frequent intervals (MacCallum and Juel-Jensen, 1966).

If this treatment is given at the start then the attack may be shortened to 3–4 days. Apart from measures designed to avert a pyrexia (such as salicylates) there is no way of preventing further attacks. The established cold sore may be treated with any mild local antiseptic preparation. A popular method is to dab it with surgical spirit two or three times per day.

4. Herpes Zoster

Herpes zoster is caused by the chickenpox (varicella) virus. It is described briefly here because it is quite often seen on the face. Herpes zoster affects adults who have had chickenpox in the past and who have circulating antibodies to the varicella virus. The causative agent goes into a period of 'eclipse' in the posterior root ganglia and an as-yet-undiscovered precipitating event causes the virus to emerge and migrate along the sensory nerves issuing from the particular root ganglion. The rash of 'shingles' is then produced in the appropriate dermatome. Some of the 'precipitating events' include malignant disease affecting the vertebrae or spinal cord and injury to these anatomical sites, but in the majority of cases herpes zoster appears for no apparent reason.

Clinical Appearance. The trigeminal ganglion of the fifth cranial nerve may be the site of the latent infection and the commonest site for facial involvement is in the area of the ophthalmic branch of the fifth nerve. Occasionally the mandibular or maxillary branches are affected but this is much less common.

Ophthalmic zoster is a most uncomfortable and unpleasant disorder (*Plate* 10A). The area of involvement includes the conjunctiva, the upper lid and the forehead over the affected eye. Pain and swelling occur early and then after a few days the typical vesicles occur, to be followed by pustules and then crusts. The disorder lasts approximately 10–14 days and is accompanied by a mild pyrexia and malaise initially. Sequelae include ophthalmic disorders such as corneal opacities, scarring of the eyelids with deformity and severe post-herpetic neuralgia.

Treatment

Usually the most appropriate treatment consists of making the patient comfortable with bland applications and by giving analgesics when

required. It has been suggested that treatment with systemic corticosteroids will help prevent post-herpetic neuralgia (Eaglestein et al.,
1970). These authors demonstrated that there was a small but significant advantage in treating patients over the age of 60 suffering from
herpes zoster with systemic steroids. More recently it has been demonstrated that 5–40 per cent idoxuridine (5-IDU) in DMSO used
topically cuts the length of illness markedly (Juel-Jensen et al.,
1970).

5. Vaccinia

Vaccinia rarely affects the face save in 'eczema vaccinatum' when a
patient with atopic dermatitis becomes accidentally vaccinated or
contacts someone with a vaccination. However, it is mentioned here
because accidental infection of the face is sometimes seen (*Plate* 10B)
and may cause difficulty in diagnosis unless the possibility is appreciated.

FUNGAL INFECTIONS

Ringworm Infections

a. Tinea Barbae

Ringworm of the beard area is not often seen now though apparently
used to be very much more common. The infecting organism may be
Trichophyton mentagrophytes or *T. rubrum*. Less commonly, other species
may be involved including species which usually infect an animal host.
    Clinical Appearance. This is fundamentally an infection of the follicle
and this may be apparent clinically in the appearance of the eruption
(*Plate* 11A). The condition may be papular and pustular and look like
acne in areas. There is usually accompanying erythema, scaling and
some swelling. If left untreated the disease persists and is punctuated by
episodes of acute inflammation. It may lead to a patchy loss of beard
hair.

b. Glabrous Ringworm of Face or Neck

This is identical with ringworm of the glabrous skin elsewhere and the
involved sites are annular or circinate (*Fig.* 54). Cattle ringworm
(*T. verrucosum*) may affect the forehead, temple or cheek of herdsmen
or milkmaids as a result of contact with cows during milking. Since the
advent of the electric milking machine this has become less common.
The inflammation occurring in animal ringworm is much more acute
than that seen in the more usual variety due to the human pathogens.
Children seem to be quite commonly affected by ringworm involving
the face and the microsporon species often seem to be the responsible
dermatophytes.

c. Kerion

This is the term applied to a severe fungus infection characterized by swelling, pus formation and eventual scarring. It is usually due to infection by animal ringworm species but it has been recorded as being caused by *T. rubrum* infections as well.

d. Steroid aggravated ringworm

Under the term 'tinea incognito', Ive and Marks (1968) described patients with ringworm in whom there were quite unusual features due to modification by the application of potent topical corticosteroids.

When such topical corticosteroids as betamethasone 17-valerate, fluocinolone acetonide or triamcinolone acetonide are applied to an area of ringworm the redness and the scaling decrease. This eczematous component of ringworm normally has the effect of limiting the extent of the infection and when it is 'dampened down' by the corticosteroids the ringworm tends to spread and lose its usual appearance. It is very easy to be misled in this way over facial ringworm (*Plate* 11B). The reddening of the face sometimes gives rise to a mistaken diagnosis of rosacea and fruitless treatment with tetracyclines. A definite edge to the rash should provide a clue as to its nature.

Diagnosis of the Ringworm Infections

The diagnosis of a ringworm infection may be sustained by finding the fungal mycelial fragments in scale from the affected area. The scale may be examined after clearing in 10 per cent KOH, or by skin surface biopsy (Marks and Dawber, 1972). This latter method employs a rapidly bonding cyano-acrylate adhesive, and simplifies the search for the micro-organism. In the skin surface biopsies it can be seen that there is a vast amount of ringworm mycelium present in the scale of tinea incognito (*Fig.* 55).

Treatment

Where the infection is extremely limited the topical use of keratolytic and antifungal preparations is adequately effective. As undiluted Whitfield's ointment may be irritant, especially on the face, half-strength Whitfield's ointment should be prescribed as this appears equally effective. Undecenoic acid, chlorphenesin and tolnaftate preparations appear to be slightly less effective. Newer preparations containing clotrimazole (Canestan, Bayer) and miconazole (Daktarin, Janssen) are quite effective. Where the ringworm has not responded to topical therapy, is recurrent or is extensive then griseofulvin should be given. This antibiotic should be given in a dose of 250 mg twice or three times per day to adults for 4–6 weeks. A correspondingly smaller dose should be given to children.

Pityriasis Versicolor

This is a mild yeast-type of infection of the stratum corneum. It is caused by *Malassezia furfur*. It is probably part of the normal skin flora and assumes a disease role only if and when the conditions are favourable. It is more common in warmer climates. Although most often seen on the trunk pityriasis versicolor is sometimes seen on the face and neck.

Clinical Appearance. The hallmark of the infection is the presence of well-marginated, round, finely scaling patches. The patches may be slightly pink or are depigmented compared to the surrounding skin (*Fig.* 56). The *differential diagnosis* includes conditions in which depigmented macules are seen, such as pityriasis alba (frequently seen on the face in children), vitiligo and leprosy (in those who have resided outside Europe). The *diagnosis* is confirmed by the finding of the characteristic spores and tangled mycelium in KOH preparations or skin surface biopsy.

Treatment

Dabbing the affected areas with a solution of 20 per cent sodium thiosulphate in water twice daily for 6 weeks is often effective. Other treatments include (*a*) the use of selenium sulphide suspension (Selsun, Abbott) which is painted on and left there overnight (this may be irritant on the face, where it should not be applied); and (*b*) the use of half-strength Whitfield's ointment twice daily for 6 weeks (this can also produce primary irritation of the skin). Clotrimazole and miconazole preparations are quite effective.

Candidiasis (Moniliasis)

Candida albicans is a yeast type of fungus that is found normally in the mouth or at the anal margin of 31 per cent of the infant population (Beare et al., 1968), and as part of the flora in 22 per cent of the normal adult population. It is a frequent opportunistic invader of diseased tissue and therefore it can be difficult on occasions to know whether or not its presence is aetiologically important.

It is more often considered to be a cause of inflammatory disorders of the buccal mucosa than of the glabrous skin. However, there are two situations that will be mentioned here in relationship to candidiasis.

a. Angular Cheilitis

The maceration, fissuring and soreness that may be seen at the angles of the mouth in edentulous elderly patients may in part be due to the candida organism. However, the part played by inadequately fitting dentures and facial tissues that have lost their normal tone has been stressed by some (Turrell, 1967).

The condition is certainly a difficult one to treat and the application of anticandidal preparations is frequently unhelpful. The elimination of the tissue fold at the corner of the mouth by one means or another is possibly more relevant.

b. Candidal Granuloma and Chronic Mucocutaneous Candidiasis
This is a persistent and severe infection of the entire skin thickness (not merely the horny layer) with the candida organism.

It is often an infection of the skin of the face and/or scalp. Infants and young children are mostly affected. It is certainly uncommon but it seems to be increasingly recognized and recently considerable attention has been devoted to the reasons for the development of these lesions. Candidal granuloma in chronic mucocutaneous candidiasis only develops in those with some deficiency in the host defences. In the majority of cases the immunological fault is unknown but in some an epithelial defect concerning the way that iron is handled may play some role (Higgs and Wells, 1972). Other patients have hypoparathyroidism or pseudohypoparathyroidism, although the way that the underlying metabolic fault is responsible for the persistence of the candidiasis is unknown. In another group of patients persistent candidal infection is associated with a thymoma (Montes et al., 1972). For a more detailed treatment of this subject the reader is referred to Higgs and Wells (1973).

Clinical Appearance. The area involved is often the scalp and adjoining temple. The affected site is swollen, crusted and may have sinuses draining pus. The involved area gradually extends and the disease may end fatally.

Treatment is (*a*) *Local* with débridement and curettage and local anticandidal drugs such as nystatin, amphotericin B and pimaricin, (*b*) *Systemic* with infusions of amphotericin B, and maybe the use of some of the newer compounds such as 5-fluorocytosine or clotrimazole.

REFERENCES

Baringer J. R. and Swoveland P. (1973) Recovery of herpes simplex virus from human trigeminal ganglions. *N. Engl. J. Med.* **288**, 648.

Bastian F. O., Rabson A. S., Yee C. L. and Tralka T. S. (1972) Herpes virus hominis isolation from human trigeminal ganglion. *Science* **178**, 306.

Beare J. M., Cheeseman E. A. and Mackenzie D. W. R. (1968) The association between *C. albicans* and lesions of seborrhoeic eczema. *Br. J. Dermatol.* **80**, 675.

Beutner E. H., Chorzelski T. P. and Jordan R. E. (1970) *Autosensitisation in Pemphigus and Bullous Pemphigoid.* Springfield, Ill., Thomas.

British Medical Journal (1972) Leader. **2**, 548.

Connor B. L. (1972) Impetigo contagiosa in the United Kingdom. *Br. J. Dermatol.* **86**, Suppl. 8, 48.

Davies M., Fulgham D. D. and Taplin D. (1968) The value of neomycin in a neomycin steroid cream. *JAMA* **203**, 298.

De Oreo G. A., Johnson H. H. and Binkley G. W. (1956) An eczematous reaction associated with molluscum contagiosum. *Arch. Dermatol.* **74**, 344.

Eaglestein W. E., Katz R. and Brown J. A. (1970) The effects of early corticosteroid therapy on the skin eruption and pain of herpes zoster. *JAMA* **211**, 1681.

Higgs J. M. and Wells R. S. (1972) Chronic mucocutaneous candidiasis: associated abnormalities of iron metabolism. *Br. J. Dermatol.* **86**, Suppl. 8, 88.

Higgs J. M. and Wells R. S. (1973) Chronic muco-cutaneous candidiasis. New approaches to treatment. *Br. J. Dermatol.* **89**, 179.

Ive F. A. and Marks R. (1968) Tinea incognito. *Br. Med. J.* **3**, 149.

Juel-Jensen B. E., MacCallum F. O., Mackenzie A. M. and Pike M. C. (1970) Treatment of zoster with idoxuridine in dimethyl sulphoxide. Results of two double blind controlled trials. *Br. Med. J.* **4**, 776.

Kaplan E. L., Anthony B. F., Chapman S. S. and Wannamaker L. W. (1970) Epidemic acute glomerulonephritis associated with type 49 streptococcal pyoderma. *Am. J. Med.* **48**, 9, 27.

Kingsley-Smith B. V., Marks R. and Elek S. D. (1967) Viruses and warts. (Letter.) *Br. Med. J.* **1**, 301.

Lancet (1974) Editorial. **1**, 1267.

Marks R. and Dawber R. P. (1972) *In situ* microbiology of the stratum corneum. An application of skin surface biopsy. *Arch. Dermatol.* **105**, 216.

MacCallum F. O. and Juel-Jensen B. E. (1966) Herpes simplex virus skin infection in man treated with idoxuridine in dimethyl sulphoxide. Results of a double blind controlled trial. *Br. Med. J.* **2**, 805.

Montes L. F., Ceballos R., Cooper M. D., Bradley M. N. and Bockman D. E. (1972) Chronic mucocutaneous candidiasis, myositis and thymoma. A new triad. *JAMA* **222**, 1619.

Poon-King T., Mohammed I., Cox R., Potter E. V., Simon N. M., Siegel A. C. and Earle D. P. (1967) Recurrent epidemic nephritis in South Trinidad. *N. Engl. J. Med.* **277**, 728.

Turrell A. J. W. (1967) Angular cheilitis and dentures. *Br. J. Dermatol.* **79**, 331.

Chapter 9

Tumours of Facial Skin

In this chapter I will briefly describe neoplasms that occur exclusively, predominantly or very frequently on facial skin and discuss the differential diagnosis of facial skin tumours. It should be remembered that the face is a particular target for solar damage and neoplasms that occur after prolonged exposure to ultraviolet light are especially common on the face. In addition, the large numbers of well-developed hair follicles and sebaceous glands also influence the type of lesion seen in this region.

NEOPLASMS AND HAMARTOMATA ORIGINATING IN EPITHELIAL STRUCTURES

Seborrhoeic Keratoses (Seborrhoeic Warts)
Like barnacles on a rusting ship, these common and benign tumours accumulate on skin with increasing age and exposure to the elements. They can occur virtually anywhere on the skin but are frequently found on the upper trunk, backs of the hands and face. They are commonly seen on the temples, forehead and preauricular regions. On the face they are in general less 'warty' and thickened than on the trunk (*Fig.* 57). Seborrhoeic keratoses are usually fawn or a shade of brown. As they are frequently 'non-warty' and brown they should be distinguished from other flat pigmented lesions such as senile lentigo, lentigo maligna or pigmented basal cell epithelioma. Ordinary lentigines are completely flat and uniform in colour. Patients with lentigo maligna give a history of a gradually extending and darkening lesion (*see below*). It is often variegate and may be slightly thickened in places.

Histopathology. Seborrhoeic keratoses consist of keratinocytes of varying immaturity. In places small clusters of cells start to keratinize and form horny cysts. In other areas they are small and basophilic, showing little tendency to differentiate. The whole lesion may appear 'stuck on', i.e. above the general epidermal level (*Fig.* 58). There is regular papillomatosis and the surface is regularly 'spiky' giving the warty appearance. These lesions show a wide variety of appearances, especially when irritated or infected.

Treatment

If there are only one or a few lesions, it is reasonable to attempt their permanent removal by excision or by curettage and light diathermy of the base. If there are numerous seborrhoeic keratoses, a less active approach is required. Occasionally the application of 2–5 per cent concentrations of salicylic acid in simple ointment used twice daily will succeed in flattening the lesions and making them cosmetically acceptable.

Inverted Follicular Keratosis

Under this title Helwig (1954) described an uncommon crateriform lesion occurring predominantly on the face and around the nose, particularly in adults. These lesions are probably a type of seborrhoeic wart (Sim Davis et al., 1975). Essentially, they consist of benign epithelial masses which show some attempt at a type of horn formation and have histological characteristics of an irritated seborrhoeic wart (*Fig.* 59). There is a central horny plug although the major part of the abnormal epithelium is below the general level of the epidermis. They are rarely recognized prior to their removal.

Epidermal Naevus (Naevus Verrucosus) and Naevus Sebaceus of Jadassohn

These lesions are benign inappropriate proliferations of various admixtures of warty epidermal hyperplasia and abnormally situated enlarged sebaceous glands, eccrine and apocrine sweat ducts and glands. They appear to be congenital malformations and are classified as hamartomata. If the sebaceous element predominates, the lesion is known as 'naevus sebaceus', but there is no fundamental difference between this variety and 'purer' epidermal lesions. Wilson-Jones and Heyl (1970) reviewed these lesions and the reader is referred to this article for a more detailed consideration. Warty epidermal lesions can occur anywhere on the body surface but are frequently found on the side of the face or the forehead as well as the scalp. The more sebaceous lesions seem to occur predominantly on the scalp. Either they are noted at birth or they arise shortly afterwards. They gradually enlarge for a short time and then become static. In some cases they give rise to a benign adnexal tumour, such as a syringocystadenoma papilliferum; occasionally a basal cell epithelioma occurs.

Treatment

This is by surgical removal if at all possible.

Syringomata

These are benign sweat gland tumours. They are virtually always multiple and occur predominantly on the face. They are generally seen on the eyelids or on the upper cheeks and neck. Occasionally, they have a much wider distribution and develop very rapidly; they are then known by the French title '*hidradenomes éruptifs*'. Nissen and Marks (1974) found that of the 35 cases of syringomata they studied all had lesions on the face while 70 per cent had lesions on the limbs and trunk.

Syringomata are small (2–4 mm diameter), skin-coloured, white or occasionally pink lesions (*Plate* 12A). On the limbs and lower abdomen they may look strikingly lichenoid and indeed the condition is not infrequently mistaken for lichen planus when distributed in these areas. They are generally asymptomatic and only troublesome by virtue of their appearance. (Syringomata are more common in women.)

Histopathology. Even the amateur should be easily able to distinguish this lesion. In the upper and mid dermis there are small irregular tubules and cysts (often of a characteristic comma shape). These are lined by a double row of cuboidal basophilic cells. Sometimes the cysts contain an amorphous material and at others the contents consist of concentric lamellae of keratin (*Plate* 12B). There has been considerable discussion in the past concerning the derivation of these lesions. The consensus of opinion is that they are of apocrine origin, but the study in which the author was concerned suggested that they might be derived from primitive cells which can also show differentiation towards hair follicle structures.

Treatment

None is effective. If particular lesions are the cause of complaint, destruction by cautery can be tried but generally speaking the scarring produced is worse in appearance than the original lesion.

Tricho-epithelioma (Epithelioma Adenoides Cysticum)

These uncommon benign tumours of hair follicles may be solitary or multiple. They are small, intracutaneous, skin-coloured or pearly nodules. If single they may occur anywhere on the face and may resemble nodular basal cell epitheliomata. When multiple, they tend to occur symmetrically over the cheeks and may be mistaken for syringomata—although unlike these lesions they do not cluster around the eyes (*Fig.* 60). Unlike patients with syringomata many of those with tricho-epitheliomata have a family history of the disorder and then it appears heritable as an autosomal dominant characteristic.

Histopathology. In the dermis are well-circumscribed aggregates of basaloid cells and keratinizing cystic structures (*Fig.* 61). When the cystic components are not much in evidence they are easily confused with basal cell epitheliomata (*see below*).

Treatment
As for syringomata.

Pilomatrixoma (Calcifying Epithelioma of Malherbe)
The pilomatrixoma probably derives from matrix epithelium of the hair follicle—hence its name. It is an uncommon lesion that tends to occur around the face or scalp. Clinically, lesions are usually single, firm or hard, skin-coloured or slightly bluish nodules. Recently, a syndrome has been described in which these lesions are inherited, together with the symptom complex known as myotonic dystrophy (Harper, 1972).
 Histopathology. Interestingly the basaloid epithelium in these tumours undergoes a special kind of necrosis, eventual calcification and even ossification. The cells in the calcified tissue can still be identified and are known as 'ghost cells' (*Fig.* 62).

Treatment
This is by excision.

Sebaceous Gland Neoplasms
True neoplasms of the sebaceous glands are very rare. A true sebaceous gland adenoma does occur but is very uncommon when compared to senile *sebaceous gland hypertrophy*. The cause of this latter condition is quite mysterious, but results in the appearance of a number of small orange-yellow intracutaneous nodules around the nose, cheeks and chin particularly.
 Histopathology. Enormously enlarged sebaceous gland lobules are evident quite high up in the dermis (*Fig.* 63).

Trichofolliculoma and Folliculoma
These are uncommon hamartomatous lesions of hair follicle epithelium which occur predominantly on the face as single intracutaneous nodules. The abnormal epithelium may mimic or caricature ordinary follicular structures.

Cylindroma ('Turban Tumours')
This is a benign neoplasm of sweat gland epithelium. The condition is uncommon and the tumours are mostly seen as multiple nodules that occur on the scalp. They are frequently inherited as a dominant characteristic.

Histopathology. The tumours consist of oval and rounded dermal aggregates of basaloid cells amongst which may also be found larger and more eosinophilic cells (*Fig.* 64). The surrounding connective tissue often has a pink hyaline quality and may also be seen in certain other sweat gland tumours.

Syringocystadenoma Papilliferum

This is another rare sweat gland tumour. It appears to be of apocrine origin and predominantly occurs on the scalp or in women in the perigenital area. It is usually a single skin-coloured nodule with a 'pore' at the apex or may appear 'frond-like' initially.

Histopathology. It also consists of two cell types and has a rather characteristic villous or 'frond'-like arrangement. There are also a large number of plasma cells present.

Hidrocystoma

This is another uncommon anomaly of apocrine structures that occurs almost exclusively on the face. It usually consists of a solitary bluish cystic structure, which may fluctuate in size depending on the ambient temperature. It is due to cystic dilatation of apocrine ducts, either from a congenital malformation or from obstruction due to some other cause. It has been said to occur more frequently in 'washerwomen'.

MALIGNANT EPITHELIAL TUMOURS

Basal Cell Carcinoma (Basal Cell Epithelioma, Rodent Ulcer, BCC)
This must be the most common malignant tumour of man. It affects Caucasians predominantly and is especially common in individuals who have been exposed to the sun over prolonged periods of time.

It is particularly common, for example, in those with fair complexions in Australia, South Africa or the southern United States (*see* Chapter 7). Multiple basal cell carcinomata are also seen in the condition known as the basal cell naevus syndrome (Gorlin et al., 1963) in which palmar pits, CNS tumours, mandibular cysts and other bony abnormalities may occur. An increased incidence of BCC is seen in patients who have ingested arsenic over many years. They also arise in areas of previous X-ray therapy. They commonly occur on the face, although they are also common on other hairy sites. It is not unusual for a patient to have two or more lesions simultaneously, especially in those who have experienced severe solar damage to the skin. Although more common in the elderly, BCC may also be seen in young adults.

Clinical Appearance. Several types are recognized: Nodulocystic, ulcerative, superficial, morphoeic and pigmented.

The *nodulocystic type* consists of a firm or gelatinous greyish or pearly nodule (*Plate* 13A). This sort is notoriously slow growing and because of this and the ease with which it is removed has the best prognosis. If these nodules ulcerate, they do not differ much from the *ulcerative type*. These lesions form superficial ulcers, whose base is covered by a greyish slough and whose margins are often characteristically 'rolled' and 'pearly' (*Plate* 13B). If these lesions affect the perinasal or periauricular area, they may be difficult to eradicate and may cause very unpleasant destruction of areas on the face. *Superficial BCC* consists of lesions which are not infrequently multiple and are more often found on the trunk than on the face. They form pink, slightly raised, scaly, irregular macules. Often the margin has a very thin but definitely rolled pearly edge. The *morphoeic type* of lesion consists of an indurated, firm, often-depressed plaque or patch. There may be little in the way of surface change and they are infamous for the difficulties they cause in diagnosis. Their extent, both laterally and in depth, may be difficult to define so that the danger is in their inadequate removal. *Pigmented BCC* is really no more than a brown/black variant of the nodulocystic type. They are not uncommonly misdiagnosed as melanocytic lesions of one sort or another (*Plate* 14A).

Histopathology. Basically all types consist of irregular clumps, columns and variously shaped aggregates of small basophilic cells (*Fig.* 65).

There is varying stromal reaction with fibrosis which is particularly evident in morphoeic BCC. The cells at the margin of the clumps are often orientated perpendicularly to the tumour lobules giving an appearance of 'palisading'. There is usually a degree of mucoid degeneration in the tumour. This is present either within the tumour lobules or more consistently at the margins of the lobules. It results in separation of the basaloid cells from the fibrous stroma in routinely prepared histological sections. The tumour lobules may have a very 'organized' look to them and on occasions appear to emulate pilar structures. This type of arrangement is associated with the least malignant potential.

Treatment
Treatment is as follows.

a. Surgical. This type of treatment is suitable for most small lesions, save those where an unpleasant cosmetic result is likely to be obtained. Generally a margin of 2 or 3 mm around the lesion should be allowed.

b. Curettage and Cautery. Small nodulocystic or superficial lesions are very easily treated in this way. The cosmetic result is surprisingly good. Care should be taken to remove all the tumorous tissue from the base of the lesion. The recurrence rate does not appear to be any greater than with any other form of treatment.

c. Radiotherapy. Modern forms of X-ray treatment ensure rapid destruction of the basal cell epithelioma, very little reaction by the surrounding tissue, little damage to important surrounding structures (cartilage or eye for example), a low recurrence rate and a good cosmetic result. A disadvantage is the necessity for several outpatient visits for treatment over a period of a few weeks, which can be trying (and expensive!) for the elderly patient. Morphoeic or other deeply infiltrative lesions tend not to do well with this form of treatment.

d. Chemotherapy. Topical cytostatic agents such as 5-fluorouracil are in general less satisfactory for this type of lesion than for solar keratoses. However, podophyllin and colchicine preparations have been used satisfactorily (Bettley, 1971).

e. Chemosurgery. There are some deeply invasive lesions which because of inadequate treatment initially become life-threatening tumours. These are apt to occur around the ears, nose or eyes. Chemosurgery employing the Mohs' technique can cure these patients where other methods are unsuitable or have failed. This method depends on the corrosive action of zinc chloride paste and constant histological monitoring of the treated margins of the lesion to ensure that all neoplastic tissue has been removed.

Prognosis

There are reports of metastasizing basal cell epitheliomata but they are few and far between. The vast majority of lesions are easily removed and most methods of treatment are associated with a recurrence rate of approximately 5 per cent.

Senile Keratoses (Solar Keratoses)

These are usually classified as premalignant, but it is only a very small proportion of these common lesions that develop into squamous cell cancers. They are usually found in the 'light-exposed areas'— especially on the forehead, cheeks and on the hands. The exact cause of these lesions is as yet unknown but in many cases there is strong circumstantial evidence incriminating such things as:

  i. Prolonged exposure to ultraviolet light (Urbach, 1969).

  ii. The chronic ingestion of arsenic.

Clinical Appearance. They are small and pink or grey, with slightly thickened scaly or at least roughened patches (*Fig. 66*). Sometimes their redness and adherent scale encourage a mistaken diagnosis of discoid lupus erythematosus. Small lesions are often best detected by palpation.

Histology. Their hallmark is the presence of keratinocytes that 'look different'. The cells are irregularly sized and have a wide range of nuclear abnormalities, including changes in size, shape and staining (*Fig. 67*). Additionally, it often appears that the abnormal cells are irregularly orientated with regard to the normal epidermis. The abnormal tissue may also be slightly separated from the normal cells.

Treatment

Freezing with liquid nitrogen or solid carbon dioxide, or destruction with curettage and cautery or diathermy is suitable when there are only two or three lesions. Larger lesions can be formally excised but if there are several lesions, as is frequently the case, it is better to use the antimetabolite 5-fluorouracil topically as a 2 per cent or 5 per cent cream. This preparation used daily for 14–21 days is sufficient. Its disadvantage is that it frequently causes an area of soreness that lasts 7–10 days.

Intra-epidermal Epithelioma (Bowen's Disease)

Lesions of Bowen's disease are biologically similar to senile keratoses, although they may be more prone to progress to squamous cell epitheliomata. They are less often the result of solar exposure than solar keratoses and are found more frequently on the trunk and upper limbs than in exposed sites. They are reputedly caused by the chronic ingestion of arsenic, amongst other things.

Clinical Appearance. They appear as reddened and slightly thickened scaly patches, which are well marginated.

Histology. The whole normal epidermis is replaced by abnormal keratinocytes, some of which are monstrous in size and form (*Fig.* 68).

Treatment

Excision or radiotherapy is the treatment of choice.

Kerato-acanthoma (Molluscum Sebaceum)

Kerato-acanthomata occur most frequently on the face, and in the same situations as keratoses, lesions of Bowen's disease and squamous cell carcinomata. Their exact biological relationship to malignant and premalignant epidermal lesions is as yet inadequately understood. It seems that there is a sudden massive stimulus to follicular growth, although why they suddenly start to grow and after a short time as suddenly stop, is anyone's guess.

Clinical Appearance. They are characteristically suddenly appearing and rapidly growing warty lesions with central horny plugs (*Fig.* 69). They can swiftly attain a size of 2–3 cm in diameter. Their walls are sometimes almost perpendicular to the skin surface. They regress after a period of from some weeks to 4 (or at the most 6) months. Spontaneous regression may be accompanied by unpleasant scarring.

Histology. There is an invaginated regular epidermal hypertrophy with a central horny plug so that the whole lesion resembles an enormous, if somewhat distorted follicle. At the side of the lesion, there may be other follicles which show a lesser degree of hypertrophy. At the margins of the enlarged 'follicle', there may be a slight cellular atypia and an increased number of mitotic figures. There are also areas of premature keratinization within the epidermal mass which appear more intensely eosinophilic. In general, histological diagnosis of kerato-acanthoma is far from easy and some would say impossible without a good representative area of the lesion available for inspection, in which the overall architecture can be appreciated. The commonest and most serious error is to mistake a slowly growing and well-differentiated squamous cell carcinoma for a 'K.A.'

Treatment

Most small lesions can be satisfactorily coped with by curettage or by excision.

Squamous Cell Carcinoma (Epithelioma, SCC)

The same predisposing features are operative for this lesion as with the basal cell carcinoma, solar keratosis and kerato-acanthoma. In addition, SCC may occur at the margins of chronic sinuses, fistulae and ulcers due to a variety of causes. They may also arise in areas of scarring (Marjolin's ulcer) or of chronic injury from heat. Squamous cell carcinoma is a common type of neoplasm, especially in sunny climates. It has a low metastasizing potential in most cases. The most dangerous sites for SCC are the lip and the ear. It is not known what proportion arise in a pre-existing solar keratosis.

Clinical Appearance. SCC appear as ulcerated plaques or nodules (*Plate* 14B). There is often a thickened rolled edge, but this is not a consistent feature. Very indolent lesions can present as cutaneous horns arising from pink, slightly thickened plaques. Sometimes they resemble kerato-acanthomata or present as rapidly growing nodules.

Histology. There are areas of irregularly thickened epidermis with the component cells showing a variable degree of nuclear atypia and disorientation. In some areas there is a variably successful attempt at keratinization. This results in the formation of horny pearls and dyskeratotic cells within the body of the tumour mass. Commonly there is an accompanying inflammatory cell infiltrate at the base of the lesion. The dermis contains clumps of epidermal cells but it is impossible in a single section to know if they are connected to the surface epidermis or not. It may be very difficult to distinguish the extreme epidermal hypertrophy at the edge of an ulcer from a slowly growing, well-differentiated SCC.

Treatment and Prognosis

Excision and radiotherapy form the mainstays of treatment. Survival rates and frequency of development of metastases vary greatly with the site of the carcinoma and with the degree of differentiation (Stoll, 1971).

Lesions on the margin of the ear or on the lip vermilion have a more serious outlook. More radical treatments are necessary for SCC in these areas. Other ablative measures are occasionally employed—such as cryotherapy or electrocautery. The results of topical chemotherapy are not as good as with solar keratoses.

Other Epithelial Lesions

Other epithelial lesions on the face that may be mentioned here because of occasional diagnostic difficulty include milia and other cystic lesions, virus warts and mollusca contagiosa (*see* Chapter 8).

Milia are tiny white papules that are frequently seen in the periocular area and in neighbouring sites. They may also be seen after blistering conditions that originate subepidermally, and are actually very small epidermoid cysts occurring high up in the dermis.

NEOPLASIA AND HAMARTOMATA ORIGINATING FROM PIGMENT CELLS

Moles (Naevus Cell Naevi)

Everyone has a few of these common lesions which probably originate from a faulty sequence of events in the embryonic migration of cells (destined to become melanocytes) from the neural crest to the epidermis. They increase in numbers and size through childhood and adolescence and new ones may continue to appear in adult life though perhaps this is less common.

The variety of clinical appearance is remarkable. Generally they are circular or oval in outline and between 2 mm and 1 cm in diameter. However, very much larger lesions are sometimes seen and are then a very real cosmetic problem. They may be flat or raised and their surfaces can be smooth or warty. Not infrequently, they have large terminal hairs sprouting from their surface. Usually they are a shade of brown but they may be skin-coloured or slightly pink or fawn. These curious developmental aberrations are thought of as static, but in reality seem to have a developmental cycle in which there is a growth phase and a phase of regression, in which various changes of degeneration take place. The degenerative changes include calcification, fatty change and fibrosis following inflammation.

Histology. They contain variously sized aggregates of naevus cells (*Fig.* 70), and are divided conventionally into junctional, dermal and compound types, depending on the anatomical relationships of the naevus cells to the overlying epidermis. There may be epidermal thickening and irregularity, adding to the complexity of their microscopic appearance. The relationship of these lesions to the development of malignant melanoma has not yet been completely elucidated.

Undoubtedly some malignant melanomata seem to have arisen from previously benign moles.

Blue Naevus

This is a variety of mole which often occurs on the face and scalp. It appears blue because of the depth of the naevus cells, the aggregates of pigment that they produce and the differential absorption of light (the so-called Tyndall effect). Its histogenesis may be somewhat different to that of the ordinary naevus and certainly its constituent mole cells are morphologically dissimilar as they are frequently ribbon-shaped or spindle-like in form.

Naevus of Ota

This is a variety of blue naevus that occurs in oriental peoples— particularly the Japanese. It is rare in Caucasians or Negroes. It is flat and a slatey grey or bluish-grey in colour and occurs around the eye and on the sclera. Naevus of Ito is similar but occurs around the base of the neck and both are similar in appearance, if not in natural history, to the Mongolian spot.

Juvenile Melanomata

These uncommon lesions also belong to the 'naevus series'. They are red or pink hemispherical papules (or occasionally plaques) that occur particularly frequently on the face. The surface often has a characteristic '*peau d'orange*' look. They mostly make their appearance in early childhood.

Histology. The differentiation from a malignant melanoma may be quite difficult. There is considerable 'junctional' activity and the naevus cells are larger than usual. In addition, mitotic figures may be seen. The clinical appearance of pinkness is due to the lesion's vascularity. However, there usually are sufficient specific histological and cytological points to distinguish juvenile melanomata clearly from malignant melanomata (Allen, 1960).

Malignant Melanoma

This is an uncommon but gravely serious neoplasm of pigment cells. Sun exposure undoubtedly plays a role in its genesis, as it is much more common in countries such as Australia which are exposed to a great deal of ultraviolet light. For this reason it is no stranger to facial skin. Clinically (*Plate* 15A) the factors that suggest that a particular pigmented lesion is a malignant melanoma are: (1) A history of rapid increase in size and a darkening in colour of a pigmented lesion; (2) A history of bleeding, ulceration or crusting; (3) A perilesional spread of pigment; (4) The presence of smaller satellite lesions at the periphery of the area in question. At a later stage the regional nodes become involved and finally visceral metastases occur in the liver, lungs and brain.

Histology. There are masses of cells which may or may not bear a resemblance to naevus cells. There is a variable degree of cellular atypia and mitotic activity. The tumour cells invade downwards into the dermis and upwards into the epidermis. At some point in the tumour it can be seen that the tumour has arisen from the dermo-epidermal junction in association with considerable 'junctional activity'. The prognosis depends on the stage at which the lesion is diagnosed and treated. It seems that the single most important pointer as to prognosis is the depth of invasion of the lesion.

Treatment

Wide excision by a surgeon familiar with the problems of malignant melanoma gives the best result. Once the lesion has obviously spread, the prognosis for life becomes very much worse and chemotherapy and immunotherapy by centres that specialize in these techniques offer the only hope of any relief (Gutterman et al., 1974).

Lentigo Maligna (Hutchinson's Malignant Freckle, Precancerous Melanosis of Dubreuilh)

This lesion may occur on any area but is more commonly seen in the elderly on the trunk and on the face. The history is that of a flat brown or fawn-coloured area that slowly enlarges and darkens over a period of some years. The pigmentation is often irregular. This lesion should rightly be regarded as an '*in situ*' malignancy rather than 'premalignant'. It rarely metastasizes at this stage. A frequent outcome of neglect of a lentigo maligna is the eventual development of a malignant melanoma with all the attendant dangers of spread and eventual death. This development is marked by a black nodule arising with the area of pigmentation. In differential diagnosis flat seborrhoeic warts should be excluded.

Histology. There are many large abnormal clear cells at the base of the epidermis several of which can be seen to have invaded upwards into the body of the epidermis.

Treatment

During the early stages of development locally destructive manoeuvres (or excision if practicable) are suitable. Later if a malignant melanoma has developed the treatment is that of this lesion.

BENIGN LESIONS AND HAMARTOMATA

Port Wine Stains (Naevus Flammeus)

Flat dark-red or crimson patches often occur in the distribution of the sensory innervation of the fifth nerve, are extremely common and can be unpleasant cosmetically (*Plate* 15B). They are unremarkable *histologically* and all that can be seen is an increase in the number of mature but dilated capillaries in the upper dermis. When the patches are extensive and occur in the territory of the ophthalmic branch of the fifth cranial nerve, there may also be an intracranial vascular anomaly which may result in epilepsy or other neurological disturbance. This congenital 'neurocutaneous' disorder is known as the Sturge–Weber syndrome. Port wine stains do not tend to disappear spontaneously but an individual lesion may develop normally coloured patches of skin within its confines. In fact these lesions rather than disappearing may become more prominent by developing hypertrophic and even warty papillomatous areas.

Treatment
In general, treatment is ineffective and attempts at blanching the area with radiotherapy or cryotherapy should be resisted. It is of more help to the patient to receive adequate advice concerning cosmetic camouflage.

Spider Naevus
This lesion mostly occurs on the face and upper limbs. It consists of a central red spot with radiating legs (*Fig.* 71). It is usually an unexplained anomaly but when there are many, liver disease may be present. Sometimes a few lesions appear in pregnancy.

Strawberry Naevus (Capillary Haemangioma)
These lesions are lobulated, raised and bright-red (*Fig.* 72). They vary in size and seem to have an intrinsic growth cycle of their own. In the main they make their appearance in the first few months of life, enlarge during early childhood and then regress in late childhood and early teens. Rarely they enlarge with frightening rapidity and reach alarming proportions. Giant lesions are sometimes associated with a thrombocytopaenia, by virtue of their sequestration of platelets. Some lesions are not 'pure strawberry' but may contain more mature blood vessel elements as well, and then the lesion looks variegate—and often bluish in areas. Large lesions not infrequently become traumatized and may ulcerate. In these circumstances they may give rise to troublesome bleeding.
   Histology. These lesions consist of agglomerates of endothelial cells amongst which are vascular channels.

Treatment
This should be resisted unless there is evidence that natural remission is not taking place or there is some pressing medical reason. It has been

shown that large lesions diminish in size with systemic corticosteroids and this treatment has proved life-saving at times when there is persistent bleeding due to thrombocytopaenia.

Cavernous Haemangioma

These are soft bluish tumours that are composed histologically of thick-walled venous channels. Smaller compressible blue swellings are often seen on the lips of elderly individuals (*Plate* 16A). They are generally asymptomatic and are mostly noticed incidentally. The term 'venous lake' is used for these lesions and they probably represent venous dilatations rather than neoplasms.

Pyogenic Granuloma

This common lesion is a rapidly appearing red nodule with a moist surface. It may occur in many different sites but frequently arises near the lips or nostrils. Its aetiology is unknown and it may be 'reactive' rather than neoplastic.

Histology. There is a characteristic change in the connective tissue which is oedematous and homogenized. Amidst this curious dermal connective tissue are found numerous *angular* thin-walled vascular channels (*Fig.* 73) and a variable amount of mixed inflammatory cells.

Treatment

The lesions spontaneously regress after a variable period but as they are unsightly or 'get in the way' patients appreciate their removal by curettage and cautery.

Pseudopyogenic Granuloma

Wilson-Jones and Bleehan (1969) described this lesion.

Clinical Appearance. Mauve or bluish irregular plaques and nodules are seen on the ears of women. They are uncommon. Their natural history is gradually to enlarge, but they are in general asymptomatic.

Histology. They contain many irregularly dilated blood vessels, lined by large endothelial cells and a variable amount of mixed inflammatory cells.

Glomus Tumour

Benign neoplasms composed of glomus tissue are small bluish painful nodules, that are mostly seen on the tips of the fingers around the nails. However, when multiple lesions occur, as they sometimes do when there is a family incidence, individual nodules may be found around or on the ears.

MALIGNANT TUMOURS OF BLOOD VESSELS

Such tumours affecting the face are very uncommon.

An insidiously malignant tumour of blood vessels termed *angioendethelioma* has been described as an advancing red patch over the face (Wilson-Jones, 1964) and the lesions of *Kaposi's sarcoma* do occasionally occur on the ear (Marks and Gold, 1966) but for detailed descriptions the reader is referred to the relevant sections of the *Textbook of Dermatology* (Rook et al., 1972).

MISCELLANEOUS FACIAL TUMOURS

Adenoma Sebaceum

The above description is a misnomer. This cutaneous manifestation of tuberous sclerosis occurs on the cheeks and around the nose. The individual papular lesions are proliferations of vascular fibrous tissue rather than neoplastic lesions of sebaceous glands.

Fibrous Papule of the Nose

Under this title has been described a condition with small pink or red lesions occurring predominantly on the nose (*Fig.* 74). They contain large cells in the upper dermis and it may be that these are a variety of naevus (Saylan et al., 1971).

Other Lesions

Occasionally *neurofibromata* and *histiocytomata* occur on the face, but these are uncommon lesions to find in this area.

REFERENCES

Allen A. C. (1960) Juvenile melanomas of children and adults and melanocarcinomas of children. *Arch. Dermatol.* **82**, 325.

Bettley F. R. (1971) The treatment of skin carcinoma with *Podophyllum* derivatives. *Br. J. Dermatol.* **84**, 74.

Gorlin R. J., Yunis J. J. and Tuna N. (1963) Multiple naevoid basal cell carcinoma, odontogenic keratocysts and skeletal anomalies. A syndrome. *Acta Derm. Venereol.* (*Stockh.*) **43**, 39.

Gutterman J. V., Mavligil G., Gottlieb J. A., Burgess M. A., McBridge C. E., Einhorr L., Freireich E. J. and Hersh E. M. (1974) Chemo-immunotherapy of disseminated malignant melanoma with dimethyl triazeno carbonoxide and *Bacillus Calmette-Guerin*. *N. Engl. J. Med.* **291**, 592.

Harper P. S. (1972) Calcifying epithelioma of Malherbe. Association with myotonic muscular dystrophy. *Arch. Dermatol.* **106**, 41.

Helwig E. B. (1954) Inverted follicular keratosis. In: Seminar on the skin; neoplasms and dermatoses. *Proceedings 20th Seminar, American Society of Clinical Pathologists, International Congress of Clinical Pathology*. Washington, D.C., American Society of Clinical Pathology.

Marks R. and Gold S. (1966) Case shown at St John's Hospital Dermatological Society. *Trans. St John's Hosp. Dermatol. Soc.* **52**, 294.

Nissen B. and Marks R. (1974) Eruptive syringoma, a clinico-pathological study of thirty-five patients. *Br. J. Dermatol.* Suppl. **10**, 20.

Rook A., Wilkinson D. S. and Ebling F. S. G. (ed.) (1972) *Textbook of Dermatology*, 2nd ed. Oxford, Blackwell Scientific.

Saylan T., Marks R. and Wilson-Jones E. (1971) Fibrous papule of the nose. *Br. J. Dermatol.* **85**, 111.

Sim Davis D., Marks R. and Wilson-Jones E. (1976) The inverted follicular keratosis: a surprising variant of seborrhoeic wart. *Acta Derm. Venereol.* In press.

Stoll H. L. (1971) In: Fitzpatrick T. B. (ed.) *Dermatology in General Medicine.* New York, McGraw-Hill, p. 407.

Urbach F. (ed.) (1969) *The Biological Effects of Ultra Violet Radiation.* Oxford, Pergamon.

Wilson-Jones E. (1964) Malignant angioendothelioma of the skin. *Br. J. Dermatol.* **76**, 21.

Wilson-Jones E. and Bleehan S. S. (1969) Inflammatory angiomatous nodules with abnormal blood vessels occurring about the ears and scalp. (Pseudo- or atypical pyogenic granuloma.) *Br. J. Dermatol.* **81**, 804.

Wilson-Jones E. and Heyl T. (1970) Naevus sebaceus. A report of 140 cases with special regard to the development of secondary malignant tumours. *Br. J. Dermatol.* **82**, 99.

Chapter 10

Miscellaneous, Granulomatous and Ulcerative Conditions

I decided to include 'granulomas and ulcerations' in this book because the face is involved exclusively in some of the conditions described and frequently in others. For the most part the diseases included in this section are uncommon or rare. However, they are often of considerable medical importance and anyway are of great interest.

GRANULOMA FACIALE

This is an unusual inflammatory condition characterized by one or more nodules or plaques on the face or occasionally on the upper trunk (Pedace and Perry, 1966). The lesions are a dull red or brown in colour, are 1–5 cm in diameter and may have a '*peau d'orange*' type of surface (*Fig.* 75).

They appear for no apparent reason and may persist for several years without giving rise to any symptoms. Their aetiology is unknown, although their histological appearance (*see below*) suggests a hypersensitivity reaction particularly involving small blood vessels akin to that seen in erythema elevatum diutinum.

Histology. The upper and mid dermis is occupied by a dense infiltrate composed predominantly of lymphocytes, histiocytes and neutrophils. Scattered throughout the infiltrate are numerous eosinophils and a variable amount of 'nuclear dust' (fragments of polymorphonuclear leucocyte nuclei). There are degenerative changes in small blood vessels with endothelial cell swelling and even fibrinoid change in places.

Treatment

Individual lesions are often excised as they are frequently small and clinicians wish to biopsy them anyway. However, recurrences are not uncommon. Resolution is said to be hastened by intralesional injection of steroid suspension such as triamcinoline acetonide.

ATYPICAL FACIAL NECROBIOSIS

Dowling and Wilson-Jones (1967) described this condition as an uncommon variant of necrobiosis lipoidica and distinguished it from the clinically and histologically similar condition of annular sarcoidosis of the face and scalp. It seems to be usually unassociated with diabetes, but is in other respects similar to necrobiosis lipoidica appearing elsewhere.

Clinical Appearance. It is characterized by the appearance of pink to brown-yellow atrophic patches which are well marginated and appear over the frontoparietal region of the scalp. There is usually slight loss of hair in the involved region (*Fig.* 76).

Histology. The necrobiotic change is subtle and can easily be missed if not carefully sought after. Surrounding the area of diffusely increased eosinophilia are inflammatory cells, lymphocytes and histiocytes predominantly although giant cells may be conspicuous. The changes are seen in the upper dermis for the most part.

Treatment and Prognosis

As with other types of necrobiosis the condition is refractory to most types of treatment. It may be partially and temporarily improved by high potency topical corticosteroids. The natural tendency is towards gradual resolution. The condition is less destructive than with ordinary necrobiosis and ultimately there may be little to see apart from slight atrophy. The interested reader is referred to a comprehensive review of this condition by Wilson-Jones (1971).

ACNE AGMINATA (Acnitis, Lupus Miliaris Disseminatus Faciei)

At one time it was thought that this condition represented a cutaneous hypersensitivity to an internal focus of tuberculosis. This seems to have been accepted with only the flimsiest of evidence; tuberculin-testing and bacteriological studies provide no support for this belief. The condition spontaneously regresses over a period of months and conclusions drawn on the basis of response to treatment may be misleading. It is much more reasonable to suggest that there is a relationship of this condition with rosacea, because of the clinical and histological overlap with rosacea. However, there is no real evidence for this suggestion either and it certainly does not respond to treatment for rosacea.

Epidemiology. The condition predominantly affects the third decade and favours men (Scott and Calnan, 1967).

Clinical Appearance. Dark-red to brown hemispherical papules occur symmetrically over the cheeks, around the eyes and less frequently over the forehead and chin (*Fig.* 77). The papules bear some resemblance to rosacea papules but seem more deeply set and darker. Individual papules gradually disappear and leave small pock-type scars. The papules do not give rise to symptoms but the appearance is unpleasant.

Histology. There is a striking picture of granulomatous inflammation within the upper and mid dermis. The inflammatory cellular infiltrate consists of lymphocytes, histiocytes, epithelioid cells and giant cells. At the centre of the inflammatory foci it is not uncommon to find areas of caseation necrosis. The presence of these 'tuberculoid' granulomata and the caseation necrosis were the basic cause for the belief in the association with tuberculosis. Because of the intensity of the inflammation it is impossible to be sure whether similar connective tissue changes to those in rosacea occur in the upper dermis or not.

Treatment and Prognosis

The condition resolves spontaneously—usually within 18 months—and no treatment seems to influence the speed with which this takes place.

LUPUS VULGARIS

This condition has luckily become extremely rare, since the general improvements in the standard of living within the community and the simultaneous availability of adequate chemotherapy. However, the author has seen at least a dozen patients in whom the disease had not hitherto been diagnosed in the previous 10 years and a high degree of clinical awareness must be maintained. It is a particular type of hypersensitivity to the tubercle bacillus which can usually be demonstrated in small numbers within the lesions. The presence of the lesion of lupus vulgaris implies the coexistence or previous existence of a focus of tuberculosis within the body. However, this may have spontaneously healed or be so small as to defy demonstration. It used to be seen in the poorer social groups and was a major cause of gross facial disfigurement.

Clinical Appearance. The early lesion consists of one or several yellowish-brown translucent papules or small plaques. The natural progression of this lesion is towards peripheral extension and central healing with scarring (*Fig.* 78). The disease is destructive and the scarring is more mutilating than that of lupus erythematosus.

Erosion is uncommon but may take place. When advanced, infiltrated plaques consisting of agminated papules are found. The disease may gradually progress over many years and the resulting scars can develop squamous cell carcinomata within them. The commonest areas to be involved are the cheeks, the nose and the ears; there are usually one or two affected patches only and the involvement is asymmetrical. The progression is irregular both in time and space.

Histology. Tuberculoid granulomata are seen within the upper dermis *without* any caseation. There is, of course, also considerable scarring in the vicinity. Tubercle bacilli can usually be found within macrophages and giant cells, but only after much serial sectioning and careful special staining. Probably the best staining method for the demonstration of the tubercle bacillus is the Thioflavine-T method which picks out bacilli as points of fluorescence under the fluorescence microscope. It is also possible to culture the micro-organism from biopsy specimens and this procedure may be important in assessing the antibiotic sensitivities of the micro-organism.

Treatment

There was a vogue for treatment of patients suffering from lupus vulgaris with isoniazid alone. In view of the danger of the development of resistant micro-organisms this is quite unjustifiable. If the antibiotic sensitivities are unknown and no other foci of tuberculosis can be detected, it is permissible to start treatment with isoniazid and para-amino salicylic acid. It should be emphasized that the treatment of lupus vulgaris does not differ essentially, as far as chemotherapy is concerned, from that of tuberculosis elsewhere and guidance should be sought from specialists in this subject area.

SARCOIDOSIS

Sarcoidosis is a multi-system inflammatory disorder of unknown cause and characterized by the presence of a particular type of granulomatous tissue reaction with foci consisting of many epithelioid cells, giant cells, few lymphocytes and a variable amount of tissue necrosis.

Clinical Appearance. There are many varieties of cutaneous sarcoidosis and this description will be limited to those that are found particularly on the face: (*a*) *Micropapular variety.* This type is characterized by numerous small pink or reddish-brown papules appearing around the nostrils, the sides of the nose and spreading on to the cheeks and forehead; (*b*) *Lupus pernio* (Chilblain lupus). This variety may affect all the acral 'chilblain' areas or, for example, only the nose. The affected zone is swollen and is discoloured mauve or blue (*Fig.* 79). It tends to be a rather persistent type of sarcoidosis; (*c*) *Nodular or plaque type.* This variety is characterized by one or several nodules or plaques on the cheeks or forehead. It can cause an erosion and may be responsible for considerable scarring.

Histology. The condition does not differ from sarcoidosis elsewhere and the interested reader is referred to a textbook of pathology for a complete description. The hallmark of the condition is the presence of the 'naked tubercle'. This is a rounded collection of epithelioid cells with only a few surrounding lymphocytes. At the centre there quite often are giant cells and occasionally a small amount of tissue necrosis.

Diagnosis is made by biopsy and confirmed by other laboratory tests such as the Kveim test, serum protein analysis and serum calcium.

Treatment

This depends very much on the degree of discomfort and inconvenience to the patient. In terms of cutaneous lesions this means persistent and disfiguring lesions only. Generally treatment is dictated by involvement of other systems. Corticosteroids have a suppressive effect which may be helpful and at times life-saving when there is severe systemic involvement. Chloroquine treatment may sometimes be helpful.

JUVENILE XANTHOGRANULOMA (Naevoxantho-endothelioma)

This is a benign localized proliferative disorder of cutaneous reticulo-endothelial elements; it is quite uncommon and affects infants aged from a few months to 5 or 6 years.

Clinical Appearance. One or a few nodules occur. They may be distributed anywhere on the body surface but are not infrequent on the face (*Fig.* 80). They are a reddish-orange in colour and hemispherical, but they may have quite steep walls. They are unassociated with any similar infiltrations viscerally.

Histology. The lesions consist of collections of mixed inflammatory cells amongst which are lipidized histiocytes, giant cells and eosinophils.

Treatment

None is required because these lesions regress after a variable period lasting some months to several years.

MELKERSOHN–ROSENTHAL SYNDROME

This is a curious agglomeration of symptoms and signs. It consists of recurrent facial nerve pareses, scrotal tongue and persistent swelling of the lip or cheeks. It seems to affect younger age groups predominantly. This disorder is subject to relapses and remissions. It is of unknown cause but the swollen areas are occupied by granulomatous infiltrate often of a strikingly sarcoidal type.

Treatment

Systemic steroids, long-term antibiotics and various surgical manoeuvres to 'promote lymphatic drainage' may be tried but are not usually rewarded by a great deal of success.

ACUTE NEUTROPHILIC FEBRILE DERMATOSIS
(Sweet's Disease)

This disorder is not granulomatous but is most appropriately included in this section. It was described by Sweet (1964) and several reports have appeared subsequently (Sweet, 1968; Whittle et al., 1968) concerning this uncommon but distinctive entity. It appears almost restricted to middle-aged women and is characterized by the sudden onset of swollen erythematous plaques on the face and neck (*Plate* 16B). At the same time there is slight fever and a peripheral neutrophil leucocytosis.

Histology. There is a tremendous outpouring of polymorphonuclear neutrophil leucocytes in the dermis and in places many neutrophil fragments are found scattered around the small blood vessels. Scattered in the infiltrate are eosinophils and the small blood vessels appear focally oedematous and degenerate.

Treatment

The disorder responds dramatically to systemic steroids, e.g. prednisone 60 mg per day. Relapses may occur, but in general the disorder is not overtroublesome once recognized and correctly treated.

CUTANEOUS LEISHMANIASIS

This subject is included here because patients suffering from it are not infrequently seen in the dermatological outpatient clinics in this era of 'the package holiday'. The type of skin disease due to leishmaniasis most likely to be encountered is cutaneous leishmaniasis, which is caused by the protozoon *Leishmania tropica*. It is spread by the sand-fly, *Phlebotomus papatasii*, and occurs predominantly in hot dry climates. It is not uncommon in Asia Minor and in North Africa. It is also seen in some parts of the Mediterranean littoral. After the patient has been bitten by an infected insect the incubation period varies between 1 and 6 months.

Clinical Appearance. The lesion is variously known as 'Baghdad boil', 'Biskra button' and 'oriental sore'; these popular names for the disease give some idea as to the range of its clinical appearances. The face is a common site for this infection. A persistent or enlarging inflamed nodule or small plaque which frequently ulcerates is the usual presentation. If left untreated it regresses spontaneously after several months to leave a large pock type of scar.

Histology. There is a granuloma with foci of histiocytes and giant cells. On staining with Giemsa's stain, the parasite may be seen intracellularly. If difficulties in diagnosis occur even after biopsy, intracutaneous hypersensitivity skin tests may be helpful.

Treatment
Pentavalent antimony compounds have been used for many years, but are not uniformly successful. Cycloguanil pamoate has been found to be frequently effective in recent years (Kurban et al., 1969). Plastic surgery is often necessary after resolution when scarring is severe.

MUCOCUTANEOUS LEISHMANIASIS (Espundia)

This is caused by *Leishmania braziliensis* and is found in South America. It causes considerable destruction and deformity of the oronasal region.

OTHER 'TROPICAL' DISORDERS

Such disorders that should be mentioned as causing facial lesions in particular include leprosy, yaws, rhinoscleroma and noma (cancrum oris) which is a rapidly spreading destructive condition of the soft tissues around the mouth. Lepromatous leprosy in particular causes a characteristic facial appearance with thickening and coarsening of the features and loss of facial hair—the leonine facies.

PERSISTENT FACIAL ULCERS

Luckily these are all rare, because they are frequently very destructive and are either intractable or indicative of serious underlying disease.

WEGENER'S GRANULOMATOSIS AND LETHAL MIDLINE GRANULOMA

Whether these two conditions are related or not is uncertain. However, the local effect that they have is the same, i.e. a granulomatous destruction of the upper respiratory tract. In Wegener's granulomatosis there are widespread vasculitic lesions including a necrotizing glomerulitis which in many cases is the cause of death. The entire respiratory tract may be affected with peripheral pulmonary lesions. In addition, about half the patients with Wegener's disease develop peripheral skin lesions. There are often ulcerating nodules or plaques. The basis for the disease is a vasculitic process which has some resemblance to polyarteritis nodosa. There is certainly a destructive vasculitis with a consequent granulomatous reaction. Lethal midline granuloma is localized to the upper respiratory tract. It is much less obviously a vasculitis. Both diseases cause a progressive destructive ulceration of the nasal mucosa which starts by crusting, epistaxis and other minor complaints but ends with hideous central facial destruction.

ARTEFACTUAL ULCERATION

The face is prominent amongst anatomical areas that command the attention of hysterics and malingerers. The artefactual lesions that they produce are usually asymmetrical, bizarre and with careful examination can usually be seen to be the results of external injury of one sort and another. Not infrequently the lesions produced are erosions or ulcers. They may be caused by scratching and then often begin as deep excoriations. At times they are produced by the application of an irritant solution (e.g. lysol). The so-called '*acné excoriée*' is not really acne at all but neurotic excoriations producing a series of acne-like prurigo papules.

NEUROTROPHIC ULCERATION

Facial anaesthesia as a result of a number of disease processes affecting the fifth nerve ganglion or sensory tracts within the brain stem may result in severe puzzling ulcerative lesions (*Fig.* 81) or in gross destructive ulceration of the paranasal tissues.

REFERENCES

Dowling G. B. and Wilson-Jones E. (1967) Atypical (annular) necrobiosis lipoidica of face and scalp. Report of clinical and histological features of seven cases. *Dermatologica* **135**, 11.

Kurban A. K., Malak J. A., Farah E. S., Siage J. and Jallad M. (1969) Treatment of cutaneous leishmaniasis (oriental sore) with a new repository antimalarial. *J. Trop. Med. Hyg.* **72**, 86.

Pedace F. J. and Perry H. O. (1966) Granuloma faciale. A clinical and histopathological review. *Arch. Dermatol.* **94**, 387.

Scott K. W. and Calnan C. D. (1967) Acne agminata. *Trans. Rep. St John's Hosp. Dermatol. Soc.* **53**, 60.

Sweet R. D. (1964) An acute febrile neutrophilic dermatosis. *Br. J. Dermatol.* **76**, 349.

Sweet R. D. (1968) Further observations on acute febrile neutrophilic dermatosis. *Br. J. Dermatol.* **80**, 800.

Whittle C. H., Beck G. A. and Champion R. H. (1968) Recurrent neutrophilic dermatosis of the face—a variant of Sweet's syndrome. *Br. J. Dermatol.* **80**, 806.

Wilson-Jones E. (1971) Necrobiosis lipoidica presenting on the face and scalp. An account of 29 patients and a detailed consideration of recent histochemical findings. *Trans. Rep. St John's Hosp. Dermatol. Soc.* **57**, 202.

INDEX